Palgrave Texts in Counselling and Psychotherapy

Series Editors
Arlene Vetere, Family Therapy and Systemic Practice, VID
Specialized University, Oslo, Norway
Rudi Dallos, Clinical Psychology, Plymouth University,
Plymouth, UK

This series introduces readers to the theory and practice of counselling and psychotherapy across a wide range of topical issues. Ideal for both trainees and practitioners, the books will appeal to anyone wishing to use counselling and psychotherapeutic skills and will be particularly relevant to workers in health, education, social work and related settings. The books in this series emphasise an integrative orientation weaving together a variety of models including, psychodynamic, attachment, trauma, narrative and systemic ideas. The books are written in an accessible and readable style with a focus on practice. Each text offers theoretical background and guidance for practice, with creative use of clinical examples.

Arlene Vetere, Professor of Family Therapy and Systemic Practice at VID Specialized University, Oslo, Norway.

Rudi Dallos, Emeritus Professor, Department of Clinical Psychology, University of Plymouth, UK.

More information about this series at
http://www.palgrave.com/gp/series/16540

Ottar Ness · Sheila McNamee ·
Øyvind Kvello
Editors

Relational Processes in Counselling and Psychotherapy Supervision

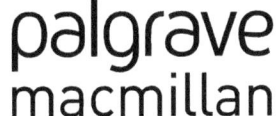

Editors
Ottar Ness
Department of Education and Lifelong Learning
Norwegian University of Science and Technology
Trondheim, Norway

Sheila McNamee
Department of Communication
University of New Hampshire
Durham, NH, USA

Øyvind Kvello
Department of Education and Lifelong Learning
Norwegian University of Science and Technology
Trondheim, Norway

ISSN 2662-9127   ISSN 2662-9135 (electronic)
Palgrave Texts in Counselling and Psychotherapy
ISBN 978-3-030-71009-5   ISBN 978-3-030-71010-1 (eBook)
https://doi.org/10.1007/978-3-030-71010-1

© The Editor(s) (if applicable) and The Author(s), under exclusive license to Springer Nature Switzerland AG 2021
This work is subject to copyright. All rights are solely and exclusively licensed by the Publisher, whether the whole or part of the material is concerned, specifically the rights of translation, reprinting, reuse of illustrations, recitation, broadcasting, reproduction on microfilms or in any other physical way, and transmission or information storage and retrieval, electronic adaptation, computer software, or by similar or dissimilar methodology now known or hereafter developed.
The use of general descriptive names, registered names, trademarks, service marks, etc. in this publication does not imply, even in the absence of a specific statement, that such names are exempt from the relevant protective laws and regulations and therefore free for general use.
The publisher, the authors and the editors are safe to assume that the advice and information in this book are believed to be true and accurate at the date of publication. Neither the publisher nor the authors or the editors give a warranty, expressed or implied, with respect to the material contained herein or for any errors or omissions that may have been made. The publisher remains neutral with regard to jurisdictional claims in published maps and institutional affiliations.

Cover illustration: Sergey Ryumin/Getty Images

This Palgrave Macmillan imprint is published by the registered company Springer Nature Switzerland AG
The registered company address is: Gewerbestrasse 11, 6330 Cham, Switzerland

Contents

1 **Introduction** 1
   Ottar Ness, Sheila McNamee, and Øyvind Kvello
   Introduction 1
   Organizing of the Book 3

2 **Theoretical Foundations of Relational Processes in Supervision** 9
   Sheila McNamee
   A Pluralist Stance Towards Supervision 10
   Supervision as Social Construction 13
   Pluralist Supervision 19
   References 23

3 **Constructing Supervision: Integrating the Professional and Personal into a Relational Self—An Invitation to Relational Integration** 25
   John Burnham and Barbara McKay
   Integration and Distinguishing: Towards a Concept of Relational Integration 25

Significance for Supervision 27
In the Beginning… Is the Personal 28
Significance for Supervision 29
Significance for Supervision 30
Ethics of the Relationship Between Personal
and Professional 30
Significance for Supervision 31
Reflexive Loop Between Personal and Professional
and the Issue of Transferable Risk 31
Significance for Supervision 32
The Coordinated Management of Meaning 33
Example (from Barbara). Mothers and Daughters 33
Social/Personal GgRRAAAACCEEESSSS… 40
Finding a Place for Feelings: Some Final Thoughts About
Our Conversation 50
References 51

4 **Relational Responsibility: Ethics and Power
in Supervision** 55
Sheila McNamee and Julie Tilsen
Introduction 55
Content or Process? 57
References 74

5 **Making the Combination of Support and Social
Control Work in Supervision** 77
Øyvind Kvello
Introduction 77
The Core Dimensions of Supervision 78
Words Are Not Neutral or Innocent 79
Supervising on How to Handle Family Resistance 80
Coping with Conflicting Discourses 82
Working/Therapeutic Alliance 88
Attachment Theory and Supervision: Building Trust 91
Concluding Remarks 93
References 94

6	**The Artistry of Stuck-Ness**	103
	Billy Hardy	
	Introduction	103
	Being Stuck. What Is It?	106
	Ending the Beginnings	116
	References	117
7	**'The Difference that Makes a Difference? A Qualitative Study of Cultural Differences and Similarities in Supervision'**	119
	Philip Messent and Reenee Singh	
	Interviews and Analysis	123
	Themes from Iranian Supervision Group	123
	Themes from Interview with M	130
	Themes from Supervision Across Region Interview	134
	Discussion and Key Learning Points for Supervisors	138
	Appendix	142
	References	148
8	**A Child-Friendly Supervision: Inviting Children to Participate**	151
	Øyvind Kvello	
	Introduction: Strengthening Children's Position	151
	Strengthening Children's Self-Agency	158
	Learning Organizations	160
	An Inclusive Practice: To Keep Children in Mind	161
	Concluding Remarks	162
	References	162
9	**Safety and Self-Care of the Supervisor**	167
	Arlene Vetere	
	Introduction	167
	Supervision and the Arousal of Anxiety	169
	Empathy and the Supervisory Alliance	169
	Attentiveness and Attunement	170
	Supervision and Therapy: 'The Continuous Flow of Our Work…'	172

Conclusion 174
References 175

Index 177

Notes on Contributors

John Burnham is a consultant family and systemic psychotherapist, with forty years of working with families, couples and individuals. He works at Parkview Clinic, Birmingham Children's Hospital where he is also director of the systemic training programmes in therapy and supervision. He is formerly Director of Training at KCC London. As well as training in the UK he teaches in a variety of contexts overseas including Scandinavia, The Netherlands, the United States and South America. He is past Visiting Fellow at Northumbria University and a Fellow of the Academy of Social Sciences.

Billy Hardy is an independent Consultant Systemic Psychotherapist, Supervisor and Trainer living and working in Wales, UK. He recently moved from a full-time University context into a new phase of practice, learning and consultancy. He is a Taos Associate and member of the United Kingdom Council for Psychotherapy. He, with colleagues, is embarking on forming a not-for-profit organization—the centre for systemic studies—to develop and sustain systemic thinking and practices. He has optimistic hopes for the reconnection and re-humanization process in 2021, and the return to and valuing of the relational and social connections we need as the human species.

Øyvind Kvello is Professor of Special Education at the Norwegian University of Science and Technology (NTNU) and Professor at the Department of Health and Social Studies University of South-Eastern Norway. For several years, he worked at Child and Adolescent Psychiatry, School Psychology Service, Child Protection Service as well as family therapist. He has supervised over 100 Child Protection Services and Nurse Services. He is the author on several books and articles, and member of the board for different national departments in Norway.

Barbara McKay is the Director of the Institute of Family Therapy, London. She is a social worker and systemic psychotherapist with experience of statutory and voluntary organizations. Barbara currently works with several leadership teams to support change programmes using a blend of systemic principles and business research. She is interested in developing networks to expand this approach and she remains in practice as a therapist, supervisor, coach and consultant while continuing to be excited and motivated by innovation and creative approaches to what appear to be intractable problems.

Sheila McNamee is Professor of Communication at the University of New Hampshire and co-founder and Vice President of the Taos Institute (taosinstitute.net). Her work is focused on dialogic transformation within a variety of social and institutional contexts including psychotherapy, organizations, education and communities. Among her most recent books are *Research and Social Change: A Relational Constructionist Approach*, with Dian Marie Hosking (Routledge, 2012), *Education as Social Construction: Contributions to Theory, Research, and Practice*, co-edited with T. Dragonas, K. Gergen, E. Tseliou (Taos WorldShare, 2015) and *The Sage Handbook of Social Constructionist Practice*, co-edited with M. Gergen, C. Camargo-Borges, & E. Rasera (Sage, 2020).

Philip Messent worked in Child and Adolescent Mental Health Services in London, UK for 30 years before retiring from the NHS in 2017. Since then, he has developed an Independent Practice, working particularly with young asylum seekers, and alongside staff in the public sector in developing services which are ethical, collaborative and transparent. He is the current editor of the *Journal of Family Therapy*. He is of white UK heritage and has a long-standing interest in working across differences in culture, and in seeking to address inequalities in our institutions, and in the services they deliver.

Ottar Ness is Professor of Counselling at the Norwegian University of Science and Technology (NTNU), Adjunct Professor at the Family Therapy and Systemic Practice programme at VID Specialized University, Oslo, Norway and Advisor at the Norwegian Competence Centre for Mental Health Care (Napha). He is leading the Relational Welfare and Well-being research group at NTNU. His work is focused on relational welfare and well-being focusing on citizenship, public value, social justice and family therapy. Among his most recent books are *Handbook of Couples Therapy* (in Norwegian, Fagbokforlaget, 2017), *Handbook of Family Therapy*, co-edited with L. Lorås (in Norwegian, Fagbokforlaget, 2019), *Beyond the Therapeutic State*, co-edited with D. Lowenthal and B. Hardy (Routledge, 2020) and *Action Research in a Relational View: Dialogue, Reflexivity, Power and Ethics*, co-edited with L. Hersted and S. Frimann (Routledge, 2020).

Reenee Singh is a Consultant Family and Systemic Psychotherapist and Director at the Child and Family Practice, London, where she set up a Centre for Intercultural Couples. She is the former CEO of the Association of Family Therapy and Systemic Practice in the UK and former Editor of the *Journal of Family Therapy*. She is Visiting Professor at the University of Bergamo. Reenee has written and edited four books and numerous academic articles on 'race', culture and qualitative research. She presents her work at a number of national and international conferences and teaches all over the world. You can find out more about her at www.reeneesingh.com.

Julie Tilsen lives on the traditional lands of the Dakota and Ojibwe peoples in the United States. She is a therapist in private practice and the author of *Therapeutic Conversations with Queer Youth: Transcending Homonormativity and Constructing Preferred Identities* (2013, Rowman & Littlefield); *Narrative Approaches to Youth Work: Conversational Skills* *for a Critical Practice* (2018, Routledge); and *Queering Your Therapy Practice: Narrative Therapy, Queer Theory, and Imagining New Identities* (Routledge, 2021). Julie's work is featured in several counsellor training videos, and she is a recipient of the Minnesota Association of Marriage and Family Therapy Distinguished Service Award.

Arlene Vetere is Professor Emeritus of Family Therapy and Systemic Practice, VID Specialized University, Oslo, Norway. Arlene is a clinical psychologist and a systemic psychotherapist, trainer and supervisor registered in the UK, where she resides. Her recent relevant publications include: *Interacting Selves*, co-edited with Peter Stratton (2016, Routledge) and *Supervision of Family Therapy and Systemic Practice*, co-edited with Jim Sheehan (2018, Springer).

List of Figures

Fig. 2.1	Relational process of constructing realities	16
Fig. 3.1	Coordinated Management of Meaning	34
Fig. 3.2	CMM construction	36
Fig. 3.3	*CMM construction*	41
Fig. 3.4	Seat/sites of identity: Creating a conversation between your personal and professional selves	44
Fig. 8.1	Different degrees of participation	156

1

Introduction

Ottar Ness, Sheila McNamee, and Øyvind Kvello

Introduction

This book is focused on relational processes in supervision for counselling and psychotherapy. The aim is first to introduce a relational theoretical stance, second to apply that stance to the process of supervision and finally to offer practitioners immediately accessible resources

---

O. Ness (✉) · Ø. Kvello
Department of Education and Lifelong Learning, Norwegian University of Science and Technology, Trondheim, Norway
e-mail: ottar.ness@ntnu.no

Ø. Kvello
e-mail: oyvind.kvello@ntnu.no

S. McNamee
Department of Communication, University of New Hampshire, Durham, NH, USA
e-mail: sheila.mcnamee@unh.edu

© The Author(s), under exclusive license to Springer Nature Switzerland AG 2021
O. Ness et al. (eds.), *Relational Processes in Counselling and Psychotherapy Supervision*, Palgrave Texts in Counselling and Psychotherapy,
https://doi.org/10.1007/978-3-030-71010-1_1

for relational supervision. Within a relational perspective, supervisor and supervisees are viewed as partners who co-construct the supervisory process. Unlike other approaches to supervision where the emphasis is on specific techniques and strategies for supervision, the relational orientation of this volume invites supervisor and supervisee into different understandings of the supervisory interaction. Central to this orientation is what supervisor and supervisee co-create when engaging in interaction. This focus directs our attention, for example, to the importance of co-creating the therapeutic relation/alliance with special attention to the well-being of the therapist, supervisee and the supervisor. Such a focus enhances both supervisory and therapeutic practice. Supervision, from this perspective, is focused on what participants are making together rather than on the individual abilities, strengths and weaknesses of either supervisor or supervisee.

Many therapists lack the time and space for offering clinical supervision to each other in ways that help clients cope with their stories and help therapists cope with overwhelming demands. Focusing attention on relational processes—that is, what people do together—facilitates the emergence of generative therapeutic outcomes. This is an important distinction from supervision models that attempt to focus solely on the supervisor and his/her skills, knowledge and techniques. Attention to supervision processes opens new understandings of the relationships into which supervisors and supervisees are inviting each other as they work together. This orientation is responsive to the complex demands of our contemporary situation where flexibility and situational sensitivity are required. Additionally, relational supervision—by inviting supervisor and supervisee to focus on their patterns of relating and how those patterns generate local realities—serves as a parallel illustration of the therapist/client therapeutic process championed by a collaborative, constructionist orientation.

Organizing of the Book

This book focuses on basic concepts and practices of relational supervision in family therapy, social work, child protection and clinical mental health work. In Chapter 2, Sheila McNamee lays out the theoretical Foundations of Relational Processes in Supervision. This orienting chapter introduces social construction and relational theory. Knowledge, meaning and understanding are seen as achievements generated within interactive processes. Thus, in abbreviated form, we can say that looking at supervision as a relational process means focusing on what people (supervisor, supervisee and client) do together and what their "doing" makes. This is a departure from traditional approaches to supervision where skills, techniques and specific abilities of the supervisor, supervisee and/or client are the focus of attention. Social construction and relational theory are introduced as a pluralist stance that refigures how we think about and engage in processes of supervision.

In Chapter 3, John Burnham and Barbara McKay write about integrating the professional and personal into a relational self. It has long been the case that psychotherapists and counsellors in training have been required to address their participation in therapeutic relationships by engaging in separate personal therapy as part of their qualifying courses. Systemic psychotherapy has taken a different pathway. The relationship between personal experience and professional practice is explored as an integral part of training courses and not separated out. This is also the case for those who go on to train as systemic supervisors where personal and professional development is a requirement of the Association for Family Therapy (AFT). Once again, it is woven into the fabric of training courses and embodied in the context, processes and content of training courses. This chapter highlights the significance of integrating our personal and professional experiences and makes the case for closer consideration of possible distinctions and connections between the two. It offers a position of relational integration achieved through a willingness to rigorously explore the dance between our personal and professional lives. It begins with an overview of theory related to ideas of integration and goes on to outline some systemic frameworks such as the Social GgRRAAAACCEEESSSS[1] and the Coordinated management of meaning to illustrate the supervisory practice examples. It concludes with a conversation between the two authors capturing some of their own thoughts about how each area of life may have benefited or been adversely affected by the other.

Chapter 4 introduces ethics and issues of power in the relational process of supervision. The shift from a sense of universal, stable ethics to a relational understanding of ethics is introduced. Power is similarly refigured as a description of interactive dynamics and not a quality of a person. In addition, the distinction between "content ethics" and "process ethics" is presented. These revised understandings of ethics and power open the door for embracing relational responsibility. If supervisors, supervisees and clients are truly attentive to the process of relating, they extend possibilities for being relationally responsible. This relational ethic invites clients and supervisees to contest therapists' and supervisors' meanings and practices as a way of influencing and informing how the therapeutic and supervisory dialogue proceeds. The relational process of this conversation is "negotiated dialogue". Negotiated dialogue refers to how supervisor and supervisee negotiate their ways forward in the supervisory conversation. During this collaborative, negotiated dialogue, supervisors and supervisees are informed by how both content ethics and process ethics are transacted as they converse with clients.

In Chapter 5, Øyvind Kvello's focus is on supervising professionals who have double mandates when combining help and social control. The Norwegian Child Protection Service (CPS) operates with a two-part mandate as described, but the issue is transferable to other professional contexts, such as forensic services and adult psychiatry. The double mandate can be ethically and professionally challenging: After some time where professionals are helping the family, the conclusion can be that the parenting is not safe, and the children are moved to an institution or in foster care. This often is experienced by the families as betrayals.

---

[1] stands for Gender, geography, Race, Religion, Age, Ability, Appearance, Accent, Class, Culture, Ethnicity, Employment, Education, Spirituality, Sexuality, Sexual Orientation, and .... *Something else that we haven't thought of yet!!*

Information gathered by the professionals helping families can be employed against the parent's wishes, for example as information for the court, where they decide if children should live in foster care or institutions for a long time, or adoption of the child. Central themes in supervision of professionals at CPS are handling resistance by being transparent, support the development of intrinsic motivation (may be developed by the use of externalizing the problem and Motivational Interviewing), and creating strong and often long-lasting working alliances. Supervisors often are the "hands" that hold the professionals when they feel being on the "top of the circle" and having a feeling of mastery, as well as comforting when they feel like being on the "bottom of the circle". In the same way, professionals should be the hands for parents, and parents should be supported to be the hands for their children.

In Chapter 6, Billy Hardy writes about the artistry of stuck-ness. This chapter is an exploration of the sometimes thorny and challenging position we may find ourselves in when we get stuck in our supervisory practice. Whenever we are faced with such dilemmas or an impasse there is not always an easy fix or one definitive strategy. The challenge as supervisors is to draw on our own creative practices. These are sometimes unusual, different and highly attuned and personal to the moment you find yourself in. These intimate spaces of learning and transformation take on different forms, responsibilities and responses. This chapter offers some vignettes [composite moments] from practice which illustrates useful learning, challenging ways of thinking, and learning across different contexts. Remaining open to the complexity of the relationships we create and re-create whilst privileging the learning creates potential for change and transformation. Stuck-ness as it has been named in this chapter is part of the process of learning and change. In supervisory relationships learning to be stuck and working with it can be framed as competence and expertise or supervisory presence held by and within supervisory relationships.

In Chapter 7, Philip Messent and Reenee Singh describe a qualitative study investigating how systemic supervision across differences in culture can best be delivered. The authors interviewed their supervisees regarding their experiences of supervision with supervisors of the same or different cultures, using Thematic Analysis to cluster emergent themes. Conclusions drawn from this analysis and building upon existing literature to guide supervisors in undertaking supervision across differences in culture both within individual countries and across regions included: a need to meet gaps in understanding with respect, and bearing witness to supervisees' emotional responses to their clients; the usefulness of a written summary in bridging language difference; the need for white supervisors to acknowledge their own necessary involvement in privilege, discrimination and racism, rejecting defensiveness; the need to maintain curiousity, acceptance and a non-judgmental attitude; including culture in case discussions and reviewing the supervisory process.

In Chapter 8, Øyvind Kvello writes about a child-friendly supervision focusing on letting children participate. There is a long-standing tradition to leave children out when making decisions about their lives. It is an important ethical decision of inviting children to participate. Themes in this chapter include how supervisors can support a practice for children's participation, strengthening agency and supporting the professionals to gain competence in talking with children. It is sometimes a challenge to develop new ways of working, which assumes the characteristics of learning organizations, because individual changes will not be sufficient to change values the organizations are based on, or the professionals' habits or attitudes. Children's participation assumes agency. Supervisors might strengthen professionals' agency, which in turn support the development of children's agency.

In the closing chapter, Arlene Vetere writes about the safety and self-care of the supervisor. She opens with Bertgers poignant words; *We are open to absorbing profound loss, hurt and mistrust from our clients but also to the stimulation of those states, present in us all.* She wrote this while working for the London Underground staff counselling service in 2001, in which she explores the double-sided nature of the emotional impacts in our therapeutic work. When we include the supervisor in the above quotation, we might wonder about the triple sided nature of the impacts for the supervisor, as they live within, and reflect on, the triangle of supervisor-therapist-client and their respective interlocking contexts of influence. There are many sources of emotional resonance in our therapeutic and supervisory work, so the key questions here centre around the development of resiliency and receptivity for practitioners, supervisors and their teams that help in sustaining supportive working contexts.

2

Theoretical Foundations of Relational Processes in Supervision

Sheila McNamee

This chapter serves as an orienting chapter on social construction and relational theory. Knowledge, meaning and understanding are seen as achievements generated within interactive processes. Thus, in abbreviated form, we can say that looking at supervision as a relational process means focusing on what people (supervisor, supervisee and client) do together and what their "doing" makes. This is a departure from traditional approaches to supervision where skills, techniques and specific abilities of the supervisor, supervisee and/or client are the focus of attention. We introduce social construction and relational theory as one elaboration of a pluralist stance that refigures how we think about and engage in processes of supervision.

S. McNamee (✉)
Department of Communication, University of New Hampshire, Durham, NH, USA
e-mail: sheila.mcnamee@unh.edu

As the training of family therapists has become increasingly formalized, focus on supervision has grown (Paré & Larner, 2004). Relational approaches to supervision (e.g. narrative supervision, collaborative supervision) are relatively new. Supervision as social construction—just as therapy as social construction (McNamee & Gergen 1992)—challenges the notion that the supervisor possesses expert knowledge, is objective, and therefore "knows" with certainty—the very features that mark the traditional modernist view of the world. From a social constructionist view, the supervisor and supervisee's relationship involves a mutual and collaborative effort in which the supervisee takes a more active and participative role in all matters related to the supervision setting. Both supervisor and supervisee bring together their resources for action, their understandings and their reflections to the process of supervision. Rather than approach supervision from the expert, all-knowing position, both supervisor and supervisee adopt a "not knowing position" (Anderson & Goolishian, 1992).

Similarly, Gardner et al. (1997) suggest that a constructionist "supervision process has as its goal the enhancement of supervisees' ability to appreciate multiple perspectives and to develop new meanings ... which can be used to facilitate their clients' therapy" (p. 219). Through conversations between supervisor and supervisee, new meanings can emerge that may be relevant and useful to a supervisee's further steps in developing as a therapist (Paré et al., 2004; Philip et al., 2007; Selicoff, 2006). From a supervisor's view, supervision may further be considered as useful, as well as successful, if the supervisees articulate their work or plan therapy with clients in such a way that involves more and new options for continuing and expanding possibilities in their therapeutic conversations (Gardner et al., 1997).

A Pluralist Stance Towards Supervision

In this book, we would like to propose what we consider a pluralist stance towards supervision. We believe that in doing so we might be able to move beyond debates among competing theories, models and methods and instead generate inclusiveness in our theory and practice.

We purposively use the term *pluralist* here to underscore the ease with which a dominant discourse (i.e. a taken-for-granted way of talking and acting) can eclipse a richly descriptive form of action and render it one-dimensional. In the present case, *pluralist* simply refers to the ability or desire to entertain multiple perspectives, even those that are oppositional or in conflict. By electing to use this term, we hope to symbolically summarize the relational constructionist argument that invites us to be present in the moment, thereby opening the space for the generative use of a wide array of methods and models of supervision.

The theme of pluralism resonates with the dialogic emphasis that has been articulated within many strands of supervision (e.g. systemic, collaborative, integrative, narrative, relational). As Sampson (1993) puts it, dialogism reminds us that "*the most important thing about people is not what is contained within them, but what transpires between them*" (p. 20, emphasis in the original). When our concerns are with what people are *doing* together, the methods and models we use become less important than working together to generate possible futures. Such a re-focusing has significant implications for our work in the domain of social care, for training others to become supervisors and for evaluation of our work.

Our main goal in this book is to propose some clarity about supervision as a dialogic process (i.e. as a *process* of social construction[1]) and in so doing, invite the multiple voices of practice into the conversation. Let us begin by speaking directly to the issues of plurality and the theme of building inclusiveness within the theory and practice of supervision.

An Invitation to Plurality

Plurality suggests a co-mingling of multiple and differing discursive options as well as multiple and differing philosophical stances. Does supervision embrace the discourse of behaviourism or the discourse of narrative? Does it speak to categories of normal and abnormal or is it

---

[1]When we use the term *social construction*, we are referring to a broad array of orientations to the study of human interchange that centre on the meaning making process. Central to this understanding is that meaning is a relational achievement, situated within a present moment *and* a cultural/historical tradition, and therefore requires a focus on what people *do together*. The emphasis within social construction is therefore dialogic.

more concerned with situated actions? These sorts of polarities are erased when we adopt a pluralist stance. And yet, pluralist activity is an apparent contradiction to our cultural mythology about professionalism. To be a competent professional, we typically expect one to be well trained in a particular model and effective in the application of that model. Consistency is admired. There is also a sense of remaining "true" to an original form. In this respect, to be a professional practitioner might fall well within a specific theoretical model in such a manner that there is visible respect for its authorship. We could draw a parallel to classical practices of music production where remaining close or "true" to the composer's interpretation is valued. This practice, of course, is contrasted to contemporary forms of music production where "sampling" allows one to mix a wide variety of artists, styles and formats. Sampling then, stands as a metaphor for a pluralist stance.

Our love affair with consistency and its associated practices of *discovering* essential aspects of phenomena as well as *predicting* future states of such phenomena comes from the tradition wherein we value science over all other forms of inquiry. Science, itself, is not the devil in this story. Rather, our intrigue with science has generated a culture of scientism (Haack, 1997) where science is viewed as the absolute and only justifiable access to the truth. The Oxford English Dictionary defines scientism as, "a term applied (freq. in a derogatory manner) to a belief in the omnipotence of scientific knowledge and techniques; also to the view that the methods of study appropriate to physical science can replace those used in other fields such as philosophy and, esp., human behaviour and the social sciences" (OED, retrieved June 21, 2018). Assuming, no matter what, that science will inform us about everything is a far cry from being scientific or valuing scientific method. In the field of relationally oriented therapy, for example, where our concern is clearly placed on helping clients find generative ways of living together, the unquestioned acceptance that scientific methods will tell us which theory or model is the *right* one to use is more than limiting. As Larner (2004) puts it, "To be scientific is to maintain an investigative curiosity about how and why therapy works" (p. 29). A pluralist emphasis (as opposed to scientism) generates the sort of curiosity that yields effective therapy due to the situated focus of participants (as opposed to a concern with employing "the right" theory or method).

Supervision as Social Construction[2]

Let us begin by talking about social construction as a *philosophical stance*, rather than as a model or method for practice. Over the past few decades, there has been confusion around social construction and its relation to practice. Since the publication of *Therapy as Social Construction* (McNamee & Gergen, 1992), the temptation to brand certain styles of therapy as *constructionist* has implied that there are some models that *are* constructionist and some that are not. Clearly, it is the case that therapy models vary in their orienting assumptions. Some theories (e.g. CBT) are situated within an individualist orientation. Here, the self-contained individual is the unit of analysis and thus therapeutic treatment is focused on transforming an individual's attitudes, traits, behaviours or beliefs. The relationship between therapist and client is hierarchical, with the therapist's knowledge occupying the position of privilege. Social construction,[3] on the other hand, assumes that the problems or issues that bring a person to therapy are emergent aspects of ongoing and continuously unfolding processes of relating. Thus, it is the interactive process, itself, that becomes the centre of attention for constructionists, not qualities or actions of isolated individuals; the relationship between therapist and client is collaborative and participatory.

While these distinctions are significant, we must remember that all theories and models are the by-product of relational negotiations that take place in cultural, historical and local contexts. When we claim that there is no "social constructionist therapy", we are not denying the very different assumptions (e.g. self-contained individual vs relational, unfolding processes) at play in modernist vs constructionist orientations. However, we must note that the title of McNamee & Gergen's 1992

---

[2]For a more thorough discussion of therapy as social construction (as opposed to social constructionist therapy), see McNamee (2004).
[3]What we refer to as social construction, others refer to as systemic social construction.

volume was purposive: *Therapy as Social Construction* (emphasis added). Therapy is a dialogic, collaborative process whereby participants—therapist and clients—actively create meaning (and thereby possibilities and constraints) *together*. Taken this way, *all* theories and models generate meaning just as all theories and models generate relationships. The question we must consider is what sort of relationship is invited by different theories or models.

This returns us to our earlier distinction between science and scientism. Using a particular model of therapy because it has been empirically demonstrated to be effective might have little to do with whether or not that model will be "effective" with a particular client and the same is the case for supervision. Therapeutic approach has little to do with successful therapy (Wampold & Imel, 2015). Effective therapy requires a collaborative therapeutic relationship that engages "a person's expectations and hopes for change as reflected in their personal narrative and lived relationships" (Larner, 2004, p. 23). The relational process and the "relationship" that process creates should be the focus of our attention.

Approaching supervision as a dialogic, collaborative process allows us to engage in the supervisory relationship in a very particular manner. When we talk about *supervision as social construction*, we are not emphasizing a particular technique or method of supervision but rather a way of talking about how we engage with each other. We shift the focus from methods and techniques to interactive processes.

To maintain a focus on process, Pearce (2007) suggestions we continually entertain the following questions:

- What are we making together?
- How are we making it?
- Who are we becoming as we make this?
- How can we make better social worlds (p. 53)?

These questions invite us into a reflexive space; a space from which we can examine what we are creating in our interactions with others. It is a space where we examine our own "fingerprints"—that is, our own participation in the unfolding scenario as well as the unfolding and perhaps shifting identities of all participants. It is a reflexive space due to the manner in which the questions identified above encourage both self and relational inquiry. That is, we are invited to inquire into our own actions and meanings as well as to inquire into what "we" are together crafting. Supervision as social construction is a collaborative conversational process. But how do our understandings of supervision (or any phenomena) emerge? To answer this question, it is useful to explore how meanings emerge.

Constructing a World

The relational focus on interactive processes, as well as the responsiveness of persons to one another and to their environment, create what we "know", what we "understand" and what we believe to be "real" (McNamee, 2014). Let us consider how specific ways of understanding the world emerge. Meaning emerges as communities of people coordinate their activities with one another. These meanings, in turn, create a sense of moral/social order (otherwise known as realities or worldviews). The continual coordination required in any relationship or community eventually generates a sense of taken-for-granted, common practices otherwise known as dominant (and largely unquestioned) discourses (local, societal or cultural practices).

As people coordinate their activities with others, patterns or rituals quickly emerge. These rituals generate a sense of standards and expectations that we use to assess our own and others' actions. Once these standardizing modes are in place, the generation of values and beliefs (a moral order) is initiated. Thus, from the very simple process of coordinating our activities with each other, we develop entire belief systems, moralities, values and worldviews. Of course, the starting point for analysis of any given moral order (reality) is not restricted to our relational coordinations. We can equally explore patterns of interaction or the sense of obligation (standards and expectations) that participants report in any given moment. We can also start with the emergent moral orders, themselves (dominant discourses as many would call them) and engage in a Foucauldian (1972) archaeology of knowledge where we examine how certain beliefs, values and practices originally emerge (which returns us to the simple coordinations of people and environments in specific historical, cultural and local moments). The relational process of creating a worldview can be illustrated as follows (McNamee, 2014) (Fig. 2.1).

This is a simplified illustration of the relation among coordinated actions, emergent patterns, a sense of expectations and the creation of dominant discourses (e.g. beliefs, meanings, values, worldviews).

We create the worlds in which we live in our moment-to-moment engagements with others and with the environment. We also inherit previously negotiated ways of viewing the world (moral orders or dominant discourses). Yet, those inherited, taken-for-granted, enduring ways of talking and acting only remain so by virtue of our continued coordinations that serve to maintain what we take to be True or Real. In other words, what we do with others matters! We simultaneously live within negotiated worldviews *and* we maintain or change them by virtue of how we interact. For example, we presume that a visit to a medical doctor is "the right thing to do" when we feel ill. It is a discourse (an unquestioned way of being) that has circulated culturally for some time. However, if we failed to participate in this practice, if we prayed when we felt ill instead of visiting the doctor—and others did as well—the dominance of the medical worldview would cease. Thus, while we most often feel

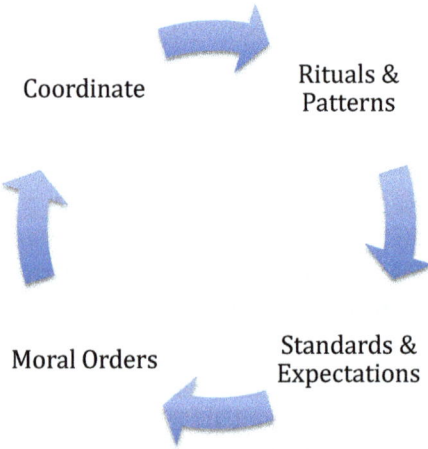

Fig. 2.1 Relational process of constructing realities

obligated to follow certain cultural and social practices, we neglect to recognize our own participation in keeping such practices alive.

Understanding the interdependence of dominant discourses and micro, daily interactions helps us to explore the process of supervision as opposed to any particular theory or method of supervision. And, it is just such an exploration of the process of supervision that we identify as relational supervision.

Returning to our theme of pluralism, it should come as no surprise that in talking about theories and models, we are focused on the discourse of all models and how particular discursive moves constrain or potentiate different forms of action and, consequently, prohibit or enable different realities. This is a liberating stance because it generates curiosity. When we become curious, as opposed to judgemental about how people engage with each other, we open ourselves to the consideration of alternatives. This particular feature is often associated with the constructionist focus on uncertainty. Attention to interactive processes positions us in a reflexive relationship to our own actions as well as to the actions of others. We are poised and prepared to ask, "What other ways might I invite this client or supervisee into creating a story of transformation?" "How is she inviting me into legitimizing or transforming or challenging her story?" "What other voices might I use now?" "What other voices might he use?" Each model or form of practice becomes another *voice*.

We find it useful to be attentive to how we might focus on our engagement with a vast array of models. Social construction is not a technique and it is not a *more pure* nor a *more correct* philosophical stance. Rather, social construction is a stance that privileges what is happening in the interaction—in the present case, the conversation among and between different models of practice. The focus is on how to bridge incommensurate models (belief systems, realities, etc.), not on discerning which is correct nor on merging different models into one meta-narrative. This is a significant difference because it positions the practitioner as open to any method of practice. Narrative, solution focused, collaborative-dialogic and open dialogue—to name a few—become potentially viable and generative ways of relationally engaging in a supervisory context. The challenge is to see a model, technique or a theory as a discursive option to be used in particular contexts and relationships. This is what social construction invites us to do and to that extent, it is pluralist.

However, does this mean that all models are equally viable? Does it mean that anything is ok? If so, why bother training professionals? On what grounds should clients seek professional help or practitioners seek supervision? Our relational, collaborative stance does not preclude evaluation. Openness to diverse methods of practice does not place all approaches on equal footing. Nor is the expertise of the supervisor tossed aside in favour of the supervisee's or client's control. The pluralist stance we are proposing simply invites us into a dialogue rather than a debate. What is up for grabs is not the notion of the effectiveness of supervision, itself. Rather, what is open to collaborative construction is the form effectiveness takes and who has the opportunity to participate in the creation of what comes to be identified as effective (and for whom). To this end, relational supervision encourages multiple resources and discourses into the conversation. These diverse worldviews are present in the dialogue not for purposes of emerging as the best or the true but rather they are responsively present to different possibilities that can potentially emerge from each. Alternatively, supervision within an individualist/modernist orientation usually follows a manualized protocol because that is what has been shown to work (evidence-based practice).

Theories as Discursive Options

Any particular discourse (or in this case, any particular theory or model) becomes a potential resource for transformation rather than a tool that will bring about transformation. A model does not make change happen; an unfolding relational process that is attentive, curious and responsive is what invites change. Within a relational stance, we are in tune with the interactive moment[4] where change might be possible. The challenge, of course, is that there are no specific techniques, nor are there any desires

---

[4]The interactive moment refers to the moment-by-moment engagement of persons in their situated activities. This focus on what people are doing *together in the moment* is not, however, devoid of the historical and cultural resources available to them. In other words, social construction, with its focus on the interactive moment, does not move all social interchange to either a level of abstraction such that there is little left to inform participants how to go on nor does

to determine which ways of talking are useful and which are not. The question of what is useful remains open and indeterminate, just like conversation. When our professional practice is understood as a *conversational process*, we can never be certain where it will go. We can never fully predict another's next move and consequently, the potential for moving in new directions, generating new conclusions and possibilities (and constraints) is ever-present. What we can do, however, is remain attentive to what conversational resources we select and which ones might serve as useful alternatives. This is the reflexive space described earlier. This relational stance has implications for professional practice in general and supervision, specifically.

Pluralist Supervision

What are the specific issues a relational orientation raises for our practice in general and supervisory interactions in particular? First, mixing theories presents a challenge to traditional notions of expert knowledge and professional neutrality. It is not the case that constructionists do not recognize expertise or authority. What constructionists challenge is the *unquestioned presumption* that the professional *should* be the authority (and that it is only through the professional's expertise in one model that success can be accomplished). We would like to suggest that the task at hand is one of coordination among models. Our emphasis is on bridging diverse discourses as opposed to making incommensurate discourses commensurate. Bridging requires coordination. And, coordination could likely include a wide array of possibilities. It could include, for example, problem talk, diagnosis and an expert stance taken by the professional. It is also likely that it might require the professional to adopt the stance of a conversational partner who does not know with certainty how to understand or make sense of the client's or supervisee's issues or situation. Furthermore, it might involve conversation about possibilities, potentials and ideals. The point is, from a constructionist

---

it move to such a singular level of activity that any interchange is capable of being viewed as a-historical and/or a-cultural.

stance, we can not know ahead of time what will be the most generative practice for any given client or supervisee.

Secondly, social constructionist theory and practice raises the question of focus in any "helping" conversation. Traditionally we focus on the past to understand the present. Yet practice informed by a constructionist sensibility places focus on the *interactive moment*—the past, present and future as they are narrated in the present. To that end, rather than attempt to provide clients or supervisees with new resources for action, the relational stance of social construction attempts to help clients utilize the conversational resources they *already have*, in new and unusual conversational arenas. Additionally, we might focus on the future, as well as on the discourse of the ideal.

Finally, there is a difference between ignoring the past (as it is narrated) and valuing participants' understandings of the past as coherent, rational and legitimate. With constructionists arguing for attention to the interactive moment, a good deal of confusion has emerged about how a practitioner can honour the supervisee's or client's desire or lack of desire to focus on the past. *Talk about the past always takes place in the present.* The "rationale" for talking about the past is not, for the constructionist, to dig into the causes of the client's problem. The past need only be discussed in as much as participants find relevance in sharing their histories. When this does, in fact, have relevance for a participant, the practitioner who sees the conversation as a process of social construction can explore how to move on from valuing the past (respecting the past) to the creation of a generative future.

Implications

In the face of competing models and methods, the tendency to slip into that sinking sense of uncertainty is heightened. The structured expectations of professional practice that have emerged as a result of scientism (symbolized here by professionalism and in the field at large by the current demands of evidence-based practice) have increased the possibility of adopting a self-deprecating uncertainty (e.g. "Systemic therapy is not rigorous enough"). Alternatively, the uncertainty that is associated with constructionism is one that invites multiplicity and thereby invites professionals, trainees, supervisees and clients alike to question their assumptions and explore alternative resources for personal, relational and social transformation. Uncertainty invites us to coordinate multiple viewpoints. We could call this *generative uncertainty*. Generative uncertainty encourages us to be responsive to the interactive moment. The practitioner is now a conversational partner who is free to move within the relationship in ways that enhance both his/her own and the other's abilities to draw on a wide range of conversational resources. The practitioner is not burdened with being "right" but with being *present* and *responsive*. All participants become accountable to each other. Yet, accountability, presence and responsivity to each other is not enough. Our conversations might be more usefully centred on broader community transformation. How might we invite each other into the sorts of relationships that effectively transform our ways of living communally together? To this end, social constructionist theory and practice would suggest that our understanding of the term *professional practice* expand well beyond the therapist-client, social worker-client, caregiver-cared for and supervisor-supervisee relationship.

We have attempted to raise several important issues; issues that must be addressed within the profession. These include questions of evaluation, ethics, expertise and training. But, for this moment, let us address only two, briefly: evaluation and training. What are, for example, the implications of a pluralist stance towards theory and practice for our assessment of supervisory effect? With the dominance of evidence-based practice, we are challenged to explore the means by which we can say that our work is successful. Rather than look to models that guide our practice, might we be better situated if we look closely at the "helping" conversation and the relationship, and construct (with our clients and colleagues) evaluative standards that are suited to a particular situation. Is it appropriate, we might ask, to employ abstract standards to a specific interactive moment?[5] Obviously, such a move would require a complete re-thinking of how we engage in evaluation and, more important, what

---

[5]See Larner (2004) for an excellent discussion of the politics of evaluation.

evaluation means. Whose standards are being used? To whose purposes? Who is left out? As Larner (2004) puts the question, "who controls the definition of evidence and which kind is acceptable to whom" (p. x). These are dramatically important questions. The challenge for the related fields of social services is to move beyond critique of evidence-based practice and instead join into the activity of evaluation—create the standards, apply the standards, test the various models against the standards. But, make sure the standards are as fluid and flexible as the situated activities to which they are applied (e.g. supervision or therapy). Participation in evaluation rather than detached critique is yet another elaboration of coordinating multiple worldviews.

Training, in addition, requires serious reflection. Can we only be pluralist *after* we have been fully trained within one theoretical model? Does coordinating multiplicity *require* initial dedication to the study and practice of one model? What is the distinction between being devoted to a model or theory and the dialogic stance of respecting difference and inquiring into the coherence of a very different view? Can we only become pluralist once we have worked with a number of different clients in a number of different contexts? How do we create training programmes that build a freedom to "mix things up" into the very fibre of the trainees' experiences? These are very difficult questions with no singular answer.

If we draw on the idea of coordinating differences itself, we might recognize that there is no singular way to prepare one to become a relational practitioner as there is no singular method for evaluation. Perhaps coordination as a metaphor reminds us not only to mix things up but to recognize risk in the very simple practices with which we engage. The risk to question what standards and what practices are being used to evaluate the success of our work with others, as well as the risk to question what will count as a generative training programme, emerge from a relational stance where collaboration, curiosity and coordination are centred. We invite us all to be pluralists, to rekindle the revolutionary spirit of the helping professions, in an attempt to build inclusiveness in theory and practice.

References

Anderson, H., & Goolishian, H. (1992). The client is the expert: A not-knowing approach to therapy. In S. McNamee & K. Gergen (Eds.), *Therapy as social construction* (pp. 25–39). Sage.

Foucault, M. (1972). *The archaeology of knowledge & the discourse on language* (A. M. S. Smith, Trans.). Pantheon Books.

Gardner, G. T., Bobele, M., & Biever, J. L. (1997). Postmodern models of family therapy supervision. In T. C. Todd & C. L. Storm (Eds.), *The complete systemic supervisor: Context, philosophy, and pragmatics* (pp. 217–228). Wiley Blackwell.

Haack, S. (1997). Science, scientism, and anti-science in the age of preposterism. *Skeptical Inquirer Magazine, 21*.

Larner, G. (2004). Family therapy and the politics of evidence. *Journal of Family Therapy, 26,* 17–39.

McNamee, S. (2004). Therapy as social construction: Back to basics and forward toward challenging issues. In T. Strong & D. Pare (Eds.), *Furthering talk: Advances in the discursive therapies*. Kluwer Academic/Plenum Press.

McNamee, S. (2014). Research as relational practice: Exploring modes of inquiry. In G. Simon & A. Chard (Eds.), *Systemic inquiry: Innovations in reflexive practice research* (pp. 74–94). Everything is Connected Press.

McNamee, S., & Gergen, K. J. (Eds.). (1992). *Therapy as social construction*. Sage.

Paré, D., Audet, C., Bayley, J., Caputo, A., Hatch, K., & Wong-Wyley, G. (2004). Courageous practice: Tales from reflexive supervision. *Canadian Journal of Counselling, 38*(2), 118–130.

Paré, D. A., & Larner, G. (Eds.). (2004). *Collaborative practice in psychology and therapy*. The Haworth Clinical Practice Press.

Pearce, W. B. (2007). *Making social worlds*. Blackwell Publishing.

Phillip, K., Guy, G., & Lowe, R. (2007). Social constructionist supervision or supervision as social construction? Some Dilemmas. *Journal of Systemic Therapies, 26*(1), 51–62.

Sampson, E. E. (1993). *Celebrating the other*. Westview Press.

Selicoff, H. (2006). Looking for good supervision: A fit between collaborative and hierarchical methods. *Journal of Systemic Therapies, 25*(1). https://doi.org/10.1521/jsyt.2006.25.1.37.

Wampold, B. E., & Imel, Z. E. (2015). *The great psychotherapy debate: The evidence for what makes psychotherapy work*. Routledge.

3

Constructing Supervision: Integrating the Professional and Personal into a Relational Self—An Invitation to Relational Integration

John Burnham and Barbara McKay

Integration and Distinguishing: Towards a Concept of Relational Integration

Integration can be thought of as 'coordinating into a functioning whole' and is often considered to be a 'good thing', benefitting both individuals and groups in the following ways:

- mixing disparate groups and incorporating previously disconnected entities into one larger entity;
- **integrating** individual and collective unconscious into what is known as the personality (Jung);

J. Burnham (✉)
Parkview Clinic, Birmingham Children's Hospital, Birmingham, UK

B. McKay
Institute of Family Therapy, London, UK

- integrating assists individual to move past negative habits, indicating a **psychological** maturity.

'The whole is greater than the sum of the parts' (attributed to Aristotle) is one of the concepts used to make sense of family and other human systems beyond the individual qualities of its individual members. Simultaneously, systemic therapists also find the concept and practice of 'distinguishing', immensely useful therapeutically (Karl et al., 1992). Drawing and performing distinctions has the potential to create different realities. For example, when we draw the linguistic distinction between the personal and the professional, we may be said to be distinguishing between two parts of a person's life which may benefit from a clear separation often referred to as 'boundaried'. Drawing and performing distinctions upon those distinctions has the potential to create, understand and influence more complex realities. Drawing a linguistic distinction opens space for difference but does not necessarily lead to performance.

A clear boundary can be a useful resource in not allowing part of one's life to dominate another part but may become a restraint in preventing practitioners from feeling that they are coordinating different aspects of their lived experience into a functioning whole, sometimes referred to as becoming authentic (Vetere & Stratton, 2016).

> *An example from John: At one time I tried to make sure that I was not performing as a therapist at home by not using any methods or techniques that I used at work. As my repertoire as a therapist at work expanded, my performance as a parent at home became narrower. That helpful clarity had become a restraint on my development as a parent. A friendly conversation with Karl Tomm helped me to dissolve what had become an unhelpful either/or dichotomy. I could think about becoming a 'Therapeutic Dad', or a 'Fatherly therapist/supervisor', when it was useful. (In the spirit of generating feedback, in the year 2000, I sent my family members a questionnaire about their experience of me as a 'professional Dad'. Strangely I am still waiting for anyone to send it back. However, I do get 'strange looks' from time to time. And am often advised 'not to try that stuff with me or my friends'.)*

In this chapter, we will propose the concept of relational integration which can be defined as a range of practices intended to develop a reciprocal relationship between the personal and professional in which each aspect becomes a living resource to the other. Professional development can enhance one's personal life and one's personal life can extend one's professional practice.

> *For example:* ***(professional>>personal)*** *the more I (John) professionally came into contact with different forms of family life that worked well in overcoming difficulties and living a life, the less I became bound by my family of origin's scripts around how family life should be lived.* ***(personal >>>professional)*** *Facing difficulties in my own life that I failed to understand and/or could not solve as easily as I thought a professional should be able to, influenced me in becoming a more tolerant, less certain practitioner. For example, our inpatient eating disorder service is organised around Multiple/Family Therapy for Anorexia Nervosa (MFT/FT-AN eg* Eisler, I. (2005), *a set of clear principles and practices with identifiable stages towards recovery. Some families say they feel reassured by this scaffold and engage cooperatively and fully with this programme and recovery goes to 'plan' (well, more or less!). When families opt not to follow this pathway, I am now less likely to explore non-compliance, and much more likely to ask what do you think might work for your family, what kind of structure do you think you could commit to? what has worked for you in the past, and what part do you think I might play in your plan? This unique plan may then be linked to the principles of the unit and a working relationship can be created through relationally reflexive interactions* (Burnham, 1993, 2005).

Significance for Supervision

- Supervisors helping supervisees to consider how their own significant relational patterns (current and historical) can be both a resource and restraint in their therapeutic practice.
- Supervisors applying the principle of 'equifinality' to their supervisory practice, and just as there are many ways to live a productive life, so there are many ways to create a positive therapeutic relationship (though perhaps not quite as many!)

However, it would be naïve to imagine that relational integration is easily achieved or that there is always a productive relationship between the personal and professional.

> *For example: 'Falling in love' in one's personal life may negatively influence how one sees the relationships that are struggling in one's professional practice. Being given extra praise/responsibility at work can lead you to feel inspired professionally, but expired personally!*

Given these different possibilities, we will also consider the contraries to integration. How to recognize/avoid each one becoming a restraint to the immediate performance or the longer-term development of the other.

In the Beginning… Is the Personal

The personal influence on choosing to join the helping professions. Before a person develops professional methods and techniques, they have an 'approach' to life, including how they consider people who are beset by difficulties or struggling to understand and cope with the direction their life has taken. In the framework provided by Approach-Method-Technique (Burnham, 1992, 1993), it is proposed that the 'personal' precedes and influences the choice of career.

A person may consider a career as a professional helper as their **desire**, (I've always wanted to be ….), **destiny** (I've always been cut out to become ….), or alternatively, they may **drift** towards it (I just seemed to end up doing this work and here I am years later). They may be following a family tradition or be the first to venture into the field. They themselves, or a loved one, may have received professional help and giving something back may be important. The inspirations, aptitudes, abilities or encouragement from others that draw a person into the field are precious resources, and it is important that they are honoured, protected, taken care of, nurtured, developed and extended. Otherwise, clients may experience a practitioner as 'robotic'; practitioners may feel 'puppet like', and supervisors may experience supervisees as overly reverent.

Part of nurturing and developing these personal aptitudes involves choosing a model within which those aptitudes can become abilities through a process of relational integration. That is, creating possibilities for the development of a reciprocal relationship between person and model in which each contributes to the mutual development of the another.

Significance for Supervision

It is important for supervisees to create a conscious narrative about the personal qualities and values that influenced their choice of profession. How will they use these as a resource without allowing them to limit the development of other aspects of self, as yet unthought of. Think about 'stepping aside' from your favourite/default abilities to create space for developing others.

Example: Stepping aside from

- *humorous responses* to play with a more serious approach;
- *being a good listener* to experiment with asking more questions;
- *talking* to moving into action techniques.

Thinking about experimentation relationally, if you step aside from your favourites, it allows someone else on your team, in your course or in a supervision group to step into that space and experiment with the very ability that you may take for granted. You may then use your wisdom to enable their development.

The personal influence on choosing a model with the selected profession. A question increasingly posed by modern-day professions is, 'Does a model work, or is it evidence based?' Another important question for each individual practitioner is, 'Can **I** make this model work?' A person arrives at the threshold of choosing a career as a professional helper with their experience of life (so far) as a major influence on how they chose *what kind of* professional helper they will become. At this particular point in the professional field, there is an increasingly wide range of pathways. Choosing an initial pathway may open up a further set of options from which to choose and so on. Whether a person decides to be 'a purist' in one model or 'promiscuous' (McNamee, 2004) with several models, a deciding factor is likely to be related to the answer to the question, 'Can I make this model work?' In other words, can a model (that works for clients) enable a practitioner to use the abilities that they already have and which led them to working in this field. If a model requires them to change/suppress these abilities entirely and permanently, then they probably will not be able to make the model work for the clients they are serving.

Significance for Supervision

Whilst 'fidelity' to the model is very important in manualized treatment, a supervisor might find the mantra: *Manualising (helpful steps) … then personalising (to the individual practitioner)… without compromising (the spirit of the approach)* helpful in creating a working relationship between manuals and practitioners (Burnham et al., 2021). As one colleague (Beki Brain) described it: '*I find my adherence to the guiding principles of these manuals is stronger when I have some individual agency in regard to how I choose to apply the ideas*'.

Ethics of the Relationship Between Personal and Professional

This is a dynamic relationship and Rorty (1991) reminds us that, '*Ethical codes are not an end to struggle, but that fairness, justice, and ethics are a process of struggle without a definitive end*' (p. 12). Each professional is likely to find themselves on the horns of an ethical dilemma at different stages in their career between personal values and professional ethics. Agencies are increasingly managed in hierarchical structures; practitioners are required to follow manualized treatment programmes; clear treatment pathways do not necessarily acknowledge systemic complexity; and professionals do not always feel that they can practice within the same spirit that inspired them to begin their professional journey at the outset. Karen Allen (2012) recommends that professionals manage their personal values in ways which put professional ethics as the highest context marker. She provides a framework and set of questions to plot a pathway through these difficult times.

Kitchener and Anderson (2011) provide a helpful ethical decision-making framework beginning with personal intuition through to meta-ethics. Clegg (2004) challenges the singularity of the prevalent bio-ethical framework and exhorts us to consider 'virtue ethics' as a framework that is more likely to generate and support 'the debate and reflectiveness needed to develop ethical responses to complex clinical situations' (p. 149).

Significance for Supervision

Although Allen (2012) proposes that, *'Practitioners should recognize and manage personal values in a way that allows professional values to guide practice'* (p. 1), she recognizes that this is not always straight forward and she continues, *'but our personal values or professional ethics may "oblige" us to work to change unfair and discriminatory laws or agency policy'* (p. 1).

When supervisees seek supervision for help with an ethical dilemma, it is helpful that a framework is used to help process the personal values and professional ethics of both the supervisee and supervisor. Otherwise, the supervisor's personal values might unobtrusively influence the outcome of the conversation.

Reflexive Loop Between Personal and Professional and the Issue of Transferable Risk

It is likely, according to Skovholt and Ronnestad (1992), that both novice practitioners and very experienced practitioners are likely to depend on those personal qualities that indicate they have aptitude for the professional work. These qualities may include calmness under pressure, tolerance, listening without judgement, a sense of humour, raw curiosity, compassion, hope and optimism as well as other such qualities. There may be little difference between the personal and professional in the early stages of professional training. At some time, and it may be different for different people, a person may begin to play with the distinctions between the personal and the professional. They may experience or name the distinction as a boundary or a barrier. They may use different clothes, language, postures and so on. Each practitioner will make decisions about transferring aptitudes/abilities from one context to the other. At its best, a reflexive loop will be created in which each area of life benefits from the other. At its worst, each area may adversely affect the other. Professional practice may be compromised by adverse events in personal life and personal life may be inhibited by the influence of professional practice. Cecchin (1993) referred to circumstances in which a person may become a 'prisoner of identity'. One of their identities takes precedence over all the others and a person becomes less agile in shifting between contexts. For example, if a person is training as a couple counsellor, they may take this training home and begin to use the ideas/practices **on**, rather than **with** their partner. This may lead them to act from a (superior?) meta-position *about* their relationship rather than being *in* the relationship. This may lead to a few frustrations, humorous interchanges and not harm the relationship. Sometimes it may harm the relationship and it may not recover. It is likely to test the relationship in one way or another.

Significance for Supervision

Supervisors need to develop the ability to actively assess

- the direction of flow and influence between the personal and professional;
- when supervision is becoming therapy;
- when events in personal life might be negatively affecting ability to perform practice;

When professional practice might be adversely affecting personal life.

The Coordinated Management of Meaning

Both authors are aficionados of the Coordinated Management of Meaning theory or CMM (Pearce & Cronen, 1980). The following diagram uses the linguistic distinctions of Culture, Society, Stories of significant relationships, Stories of self, Definitions of relationships, Episodes and Speech Acts and visually distinguishes between the horizontal (heterarchical) and the integrative (vertical) relationship. The framework acts as a scaffold within which to construct a relational integration of the personal and professional. The construction is usually performed through using questions drawn from systemic (Tomm, 1987, 1988) and narrative models (Freedman & Combs, 1996) to explore the similarities and differences between the personal and professional **within** each distinction, and **between** the distinctions (Fig. 3.1). The couplet of questions and responses begin to 'fill in the blanks' and 'colour in' the template so that it becomes a richer tapestry of distinctions and connections that might be described as a relational integration of the personal and professional, as described in Barbara's example below:

Example (from Barbara). Mothers and Daughters

This example of a supervisory conversation is informed by a recent presentation that I delivered at a national conference in which I tracked the turning points in my own family history and explored the influence that these significant events had on my own personal story and professional practice. I will outline the supervisory issue and how I use a CMM construction to co-create new opportunities for direct therapeutic practice. I will show that by incorporating personal stories into our professional practice, we open up more possibilities with clients and show more compassion in human relationships.

I chose CMM as a conversational scaffold for two reasons. Firstly, my supervisee was familiar with the tenets of CMM and communication

P	Culture	P
E	Society	R
R	Stories of significant relationships	O
S	Stories of self	F
O	Definition of relationship	E
N	Episodes	S
A	Speech Acts	S
L		I
		O
		N
		A
		L

Fig. 3.1 Coordinated Management of Meaning

approaches which created a shared language. Secondly, she had expressed interest in becoming more skilled in its use by experiencing it for herself. Although the supervision session was via zoom, we both constructed the hierarchy model to scaffold our conversations. This made it possible to name the levels of context at each stage of our conversation and to identify moments when our personal experiences were influential in our professional practice. Debby found this particularly useful in preparation for the ongoing work with she was to do with the family she brought to supervision.

My female supervisee is Debby. She is in her mid-fifties, white, English, middle class with a strong sense of spirituality. I have known Debby for about ten years, and we meet once a month. In one session, Debby talked of her frustration of working with a mother/adult daughter system. Her mandate for work was a common agreement between mother and daughter that they wanted their relationship to be better. Their history included what sounded like an oscillation between being too close, with mother seeking to influence her daughter's life, which generated some withdrawal practices such as distancing behaviour by daughter as she was working to establish her independence from the influence of mother. Mother would then frame this as uncaring, leading the daughter to feel guilty and try to repair by seeking closeness and the pattern continued. Debby named her dilemma as struggling to amplify stories of connection and hope, as the pattern of withdrawing and temporarily connecting seemed to have a relentless presence pushing this mother and daughter further apart and paralysing Debby's practice.

My relationship with Debby is characterised by bringing forth conversations and opening up new possibilities, sometimes focused on practice interventions, sometimes on meaning and patterns. For some reason in this situation, my interventions appeared to repeat the pattern of the family system with Debby pushing back at every point. We were also falling into restricting problem saturated stories unable to amplify alternatives and more hopeful positions. In short, we were replicating the pattern of the client system with my persistence in trying to be helpful and Debby's response of standing her ground and withdrawing from the conversation.

In order to co-create a different conversation, I began to wonder what 'mother/daughter' stories we were enacting in our supervision (with the family in mind). The CMM construction shows the differences in our personal positions as mothers/daughters that might be relevant to our professional activity in supervision (Fig. 3.2).

In co-creating the CMM structure, Debby and I realised that we were using different mother/daughter narratives and not coordinating in the most useful way. I decided to take a different turn in the conversation that focused on our personal experiences.

Supervisor: What are the stories of mothers and daughters that we have available to us through our own personal experience that might influence our approach to these clients?

This is the personal story I offered from my professional position: *Having been raised as an only child in a working-class mining community in the North East of England, I came to know men as providers and women as homemakers. This seemed usual to me as all of my family and friends*

	Self/supervisor	Self/supervisee	Clients
Culture	northern working class	south east middle class	south east working class
	Bringing forth resources – women are the bedrock of the family (may link me with the client mother)	Highly educated/able stories of independent women who make their own decisions (may be more aligned to the client daughter)	Unemployed- mother keen to support her only daughter Daughter keen to secure more independence
Family belief	All for one and one for all – interdependence	I'm all right jack - independence	Mother interdependence Daughter independence but recognise the need for support
	Collective women's stories	Self determination	Oscillation between interdependence and independence
Life script	talk daily	talk when problem	talk daily, usually a problem

Fig. 3.2 CMM construction

	Out in the open relationships can take differences of opinion	hesitant about upsetting others that leads to rejection	Talking and problems synonymous
Relationship	Comfortable	dis-ease	eggshells
	Relational/risk taking, relationship always stronger than any event	worried about criticism, episodes often define the relationship	Close and distant – can't free themselves from the pattern
Episode/s	dutiful daughter	reluctant daughter	work in progress
	Leaning in to talk	stepping back	Don't know how to talk
Speech act	Considerate	Guarded	Confused
	Appreciative positions	wary about what to say/share	Want it to be different – agreement

Fig. 3.2 (continued)

were living in similar circumstances. What I also gleaned was that family was everything and that close connection was expected and primarily shown by women. Any dissent was masked in favour of peace and calm. Something I did not notice until recently, was that despite the community culture of men making decisions and being the source of income, women in my family have been quietly influential and promoting independent thinking (although many of them could not show independent action).

I call into view my great grandmother who was the only licensed public house landlady in the area. I know this was as a protection against her husband 'drinking all of the profits' but nevertheless, she was a pioneer. She passed down a strong sense of what she would have called 'gumption' through the female line. However, due to world wars, the next two generations were more occupied with the family, as the men were called upon for service in the mines to produce more coal as part of the war effort. This context of constraint severely affected my mother who had many dreams that were never realised. She took on caring roles for several generations of women in her family, namely her grandmother and youngest sister. We all lived under the same roof and it is in this environment I learned about women in families.

My mother was determined that I should have a different experience of womanhood that included choice and opportunity (even though at that time my father had a successful fish and chip shop that he longed to pass on to me). My response to Debby was in this context of gratitude and closeness to my own mother for standing up for me as her daughter.

This is the personal story Debby offered: Debby told her story of being the only girl in a family of four boys. Due to her father's profession, which required frequent geographical relocation, all of the children attended boarding schools from an early age, spending holiday time with parents in different countries. Debby's experience of family was one of independence and self-determination. Her overriding story of family is one of wonderful reunions often followed by painful separations. In this context she developed an admiration for her parents and their decision to travel the world and simultaneously a disappointment that they chose to be apart from their children.

Debby remains connected with her siblings. Their conversations are currently occupied with caring for their mother since father's death, as she is alone in a community that is fairly new to her. Debby, at the moment, is trying to work out how much to support her mother and seek closeness as a daughter. Her brothers are choosing to remain distant. Despite the family story of independence, as the only female sibling, Debby appears to be stepping into (or perhaps pushed into) a gendered discourse that she should try to repair relationships and secure closeness.

This is a snapshot of our conversation.

> *Supervisor:* If your clients could pick out some themes from our experiences of being mothers and daughters, what do you think they would notice?
> *Debby:* I think they would both notice that, like many mothers and daughters, they are trying to work out the balance between closeness and distance. I think the mother would be keen to develop more connection

with her daughter and I am also wondering whether the daughter (now that she has become a mother) might be thinking about independence by creating some distance in creating her own family whilst still wanting to be close.

Supervisor: How do you think your way of navigating the balance of your relationship with your own mother might help here?

Debby: I am not sure I have got that right yet. I am very tentative about this because I don't feel I know her that well and it feels strange to say that. So, I'm not sure what to do or say as I seem to upset her a lot and she irritates me sometimes.

Supervisor: As someone who was close to my mother, I always thought that, even when we disagreed, I was always sure it would work out. I am wondering what events or episodes you and your mother have experienced that might make you confident about this or hesitant that things will work out or whether getting to know her is the start of something new?

Debby: I can't think of anything specific except that, when we were all together, there was so much competition for her attention that I often felt pushed out. I am sure it was the same for the boys, but they did not seem to mind that much. Because we did not see our parents that often, things never got sorted out. We were always going back to school or university. We never lived with them much. I guess it is a bit like starting afresh even at our age. I am not sure what I can expect of her and she probably thinks the same about me.

Supervisor: What ideas do you think you might be holding on to about mothers and daughters that is lingering with this piece of work?

Debby: I have an idea that women should be close and, as a therapist, I should be able to do this. So, I keep thinking if I can't do it yet, how can I help this mother and daughter?

Supervisor: What moments of success can you recall about your efforts with your mother as you get to know her better?

Debby: Well, I have worked out that she is strong minded and that it is useless to disagree. So, I find that I bite my tongue a lot. I have decided that she may not have many years left and that being disappointed with her is not getting me anywhere.

Supervisor: When you hear yourself say these things, what does it make you think about your clients?

Debby: It makes me think that I could talk with them about time and perhaps explore what kind of mother and daughter they think they can

be, rather than the mother and daughter I might want them to be. Maybe I should ask them what they know about one another and what they would like to know about one another?
Supervisor: If all of the mothers in our minds at the moment could add something to that what would it be? I think my mother would say that daughters sometimes turn into their mothers. So, it is best to get to know them!!
What would your mother say?
Debby: My mother would say that mothers can be your best friends if you let them.

We went on to explore what difference the turn towards personal stories created in our supervision session and the effect on the direct therapeutic work. It seemed to enable us to bring the richness of our own experiences into more creative ideas to share with the client system. We were able to position ourselves as both mother and daughter and wonder what differences it made to our conversation that we were also both mothers of daughters and our aspirations for our own relationships were informed by our relationship with our mothers (Fig. 3.3).

Social/Personal GgRRAAAACCEEESSSS…

There are many ways to think about personhood. The Mnemonic of Social GgRRAAAACCEEESSSS (Burnham, 1992; Burnham, 2012; Burnham & Nolte, 2020; Roper-Hall, 1998) stands for Gender, geography, Race, Religion, Age, Ability, Appearance, Accent, Class, Culture, Ethnicity, Employment, Education, Spirituality, Sexuality, Sexual Orientation, and ……. *Something else that we haven't thought of yet!!* It has been adopted as a handy reminder and a guide towards promoting Graceful Practice (Burnham, 1992) in many training institutions. The components of GgRRAAAACCEEESSSS can be thought of as distinctions constructed within social contexts and made by a person about themselves and about a person by others. Further distinctions can be made such as 'Visible and Voiced' and 'Invisible and Unvoiced' (Burnham, 2012). Relational integration in supervision would aim to promote practitioners' abilities to achieve an active awareness of these different aspects

<<<<<<<CLIENT>>>>>>>		
S	Culture	S
U	Society	U
P	Stories of significant relationships	P
E	Stories of self	E
R	Definition of relationship	R
V	Episodes	V
I	Speech Acts	I
S		S
O		E
R		E

Fig. 3.3 *CMM construction*

of their own personhood and consider the mutual influence (Wiener, 1953) between these aspects on how they perform themselves in therapy and supervision. All of those engaged in therapy and supervision may choose to not share the 'invisible and unvoiced' Social GgRRAAAAC-CEEESSSS but, have little choice over the 'Visible and Voiced Social GgRRAAAACCEEESSSS. Supervision can help supervisees to manage the integration of these aspects into their therapeutic practice.

> *Example: A young, white, female therapist in training was working with families with young children where parents were defined as having multiple difficulties, including their child rearing practices. The therapist was often asked, 'Do you have children yourself?' (uncovering invisible and unvoiced). She initially responded to this by 'blushing,' becoming 'flustered' and felt her confidence draining. In supervision we experimented with different ways of*

responding and she eventually chose to smile and say something like, 'You are in luck..... (pause) ... I don't have any children. So, I won't be trying to tell you what a good parent I am. I'll be more committed to helping you become the kind of parent you want to be.'

In this example, based on what was 'visible/voiced', the clients hypothesized about the 'invisible/unvoiced' aspects of the therapist's Social GgRRAAAACCEEESSSS and their influence on their abilities to help. Retrospective supervision helped the supervisee to integrate these into her presentation of self as therapist and consequently as a resource for the therapeutic relationship rather than a restraint.

In live supervision the supervisory relationship is present and can be used as an immediate resource to the therapist in developing a therapeutic relationship.

Example: A young, recently qualified therapist was in live supervision with a family and myself as supervisor. He was working with an adult family and he was the youngest person in the room. He experienced (again) that the family did not show much confidence in him, and he interpreted their questions as implicit criticisms of his ability to help them, due to his youth and relative lack of experience.

After about 20 min, he took time out for live supervision, behind the screen and not in front of the family. He shared his growing sense of self doubt about his ability to help the family. After some discussion we decided that he would adopt a posture of transparency.

When he re-joined the session, he announced to the family: In the discussion with my supervisor, who is older, more experienced and probably more knowledgeable, he agreed with you that we should be realistic in thinking about how much change we can achieve in therapy. As for me, I know that I am the youngest person here. I have far less life experience than all of you and I am probably less knowledgeable and skilled than my supervisor, at least that's what he tells me anyway! (Laughter from the family which the therapist joins in with). But, after talking with you, I think I bring an optimism 'to the party.' I have strong faith that things can be different. I am willing to work on things if you are also willing.. how about it?

Some family members were amused by this 'announcement', and others looked quite reflective. The son said, 'That's just how I feel in my family. Because I am the youngest, I feel my family, including my older sibs, don't take me seriously'. The therapist 'speaking out' about how he felt positioned in the therapeutic system due to how he was being constructed based on his **age, appearance and education**, seemed to free the son to 'speak out' about his position in the family, which was responded to thoughtfully by family members. Other family members began to reflect out loud about their experience of being positioned by others on different aspects of Social GgRRAAAACCEEESSSS. This seemed to have therapeutic effects beyond the original supervisory intention.

Taking an emotional risk in the supervisory relationship: voicing (speaking out) the invisible (optimism, faith and willingness) can open space for different possibilities. As Watzlawick et al. (1974) say, 'It's better to advertise than conceal'.

An Exercise in Relational Integration: Creating a Conversation Between Your Personal and Professional Selves

This exercise was created spontaneously with and for a student as a conversation between two selves which she named 'Student on the Course' and 'Practitioner in the Agency' and has been used in many different trainings and workshops. Here it is used to create a 'conversation for one', between the personal and professional selves. It might be called many things: 'An exercise for groups of one', 'Seats of identity', 'Sites of identity', 'Getting to know yourself', 'Self-reflexivity as a performance', 'Embodied self-reflexivity', 'Relational-reflexivity between your-selves', 'Externalising the internalised selves', 'Thinking outside your Head' and so on (Fig. 3.4).

> **Seat/sites of identity: Creating a conversation between your personal and professional selves.**
>
> Supervisees often wonder about integrating their personal and professional identities. The following exercise in self-reflexivity is designed to promote this wondering in ways which facilitate the relational integration of the personal and the professional. The exercise goes something like this:
>
> **Supervisee:** 'I feel sometimes that there is not enough connection between my personal resources and my professional practice. I have seen clients really value colleagues who make use of aspects of their personal self.
>
> **Supervisor:** Have the two of you ever had a conversation with one another?
>
> **Supervisee:** Who?
>
> **Supervisor:** Mary Personal and Mary Professional
>
> **Supervisee:** Laughing … no
>
> **Supervisor:** How about it then? How about if Mary Personal and Mary Professional have a conversation together about how they can contribute to each other's development?
>
> **Supervisee:** OK. How will that go?
>
> **Supervisor** arranges two chairs at an angle for a conversation. One seat is designated for Mary Personal and the other for Mary Professional.

Fig. 3.4 Seat/sites of identity: Creating a conversation between your personal and professional selves

Supervisor: Between Mary Personal and Mary Professional, who is most ready to speak out, or be curious about the other?

Supervisee: Mmmm… I think that Mary Personal is pretty keen to explore some issues with Mary Professional.

Supervisor: OK…away you go Mary Personal.

'Mary Personal: Nice to talk with you … (Question to supervisor: shall I say Mary Professional or you?

Supervisor: Keep the distinctions between the self stories clear by using the two names. You might even want to embody the difference in how you sit or sound.

Supervisee: OK .. Mary Personal . . . pauses, adjusts her posture and starts again. Nice to talk with you, Mary Professional. I don't know if you realise it, but I've been observing your professional development very closely for some time now. I've found myself wanting to join in with your work and wondered whether you ever intended to use me as a resource in your practice?

Supervisor: OK, interesting question. Please, move across to Mary Professional's seat and respond to the question.

Mary Professional: Thank you for that question. Yes, I have been very aware of your interest, Mary Personal, in my development. I do appreciate that interest, but I am a little cautious, well, quite a bit cautious, to let you join in. Do you have any particular ideas about how I could use you, Mary Personal, as a resource in my

Fig. 3.4 (continued)

professional practice?

Supervisor: gestures to move across to the other chair.

Mary Personal: I'm pleased that you are interested in my views. You sometimes keep me on quite a tight rein. Well, I think that some of my experiences could be usefully shared with clients. Not in an instructive way, but as a way of showing you are human as well as professional. I also think you might use my sense of humour a little more. (Mary has the hang of this now and moves across.)

Mary Professional: That sounds interesting. I think I might be willing to include some of your experiences and your sense of humour. I would worry that you, Mary Personal might take over. You know how headstrong you can be sometimes!! (Laughing)………. Seriously, which experiences did you have in mind and perhaps, more importantly, which family did you have in mind? (pause and then moved across chairs or sites/seats of identity).

Mary Personal: I was thinking about starting "small" (making that quotation mark with her fingers). The young person in the family you, Mary Professional, saw last week asked you if you had ever experimented with drugs when you were their age, and you changed the subject. Why was that? (Moved slowly across to the other seat of identity)

Mary Professional: (Sat a while) …. Well, it's complicated …. There are a few reasons why I changed the subject. I haven't (experimented with drugs), but I

Fig. 3.4 (continued)

> didn't just want to say "no" and sound like a "goody goody" who she couldn't relate to. I also wondered what my supervisor might think about it. So, I decided to respond by changing the subject. But I wished I could have responded more aesthetically, without the young person feeling like I avoided her question altogether, or that I disapproved so much that I needed to avoid her question altogether. ....pause .... Perhaps now would be a good time to ask for reflections and suggestions for others in the group about how I might have responded differently including sharing some personal experiences.
>
> The exercise shifted to discussing how Mary professional could draw upon experiences she had had as a young person where she had experimented and faced making difficult choices about what to do. This would involve sharing her personal experience at the level of process of experimenting rather than any particular content.

Fig. 3.4 (continued)

Ending with a Personal and Professional Conversation

By way of drawing the chapter to a close, we talked together about how key moments in our personal lives have influenced our professional practice and how moments in our professional practice have created ripples in our personal lives. These are some of the themes that we selected from the recording of our conversation.

> *John*: When the personal goes into the professional or the professional goes into the personal, at best it can enrich and extend mutually, but thinking

about this, at its worst, it can affect and potentially end relationships. There is some evidence that counselling training can change people and they act differently with their families. This is a serious point as there is huge emotional commitment that can be expensive in their personal relationships.

Barbara: I can think of an example where my husband said that he thought we had parented our children better because of my family therapy training. He noticed the way that I talked to the children when they were doing something wrong and noted that I showed patience and avoided criticising them.

John: I remember things that I regret as a parent that are burnt into my memory. I asked my children (now grown) about certain events, about which I am not proud, but they said they only remembered the good stuff. (I was drawing up my will at the time!). This serves as a helpful reminder that relationships can incorporate regretful events and remembering those events can help us to avoid repeating the patterns that generate regret.

Barbara: This makes me think of genogram work that we did during training. This highlighted stories of resilient women for me that I had not noticed due to my overriding observation that women were always stay at home Mams. It was only when I took the time to develop richer versions of these women that I found they were strong and influential people who were not always in the background but constrained by the time, class and culture in which they lived. This knowledge has made me more curious about the discourses of gender in my professional practice and as a mother of a daughter and granddaughters, it remains a passion to promote female voices.

John: (laughing) Growing up, I have many stories of drunken men, sometimes, as if there was no alternative way of living as a man. At aged 50, I realised that this was a choice and decided to give up drinking alcohol totally. This reminds me to develop counter-cultural ideas and promote the notion that we don't have to repeat the errors that we see around us. Seeing the effects of different kinds of behaviour makes me curious about those moments when clients might say—*'well you know how it is'*—assuming that family/cultural traditions are unchangeable.

John: You know I think I was a marital therapist from about the age of 7! In my family I used to smooth the waters between my parents and others in the family. I was a mediator, seeing both sides and used humour sometimes to dissolve violence. I was used to verbal violence which sometimes became physical, and so feel able to manage situations when emotions run high. Training confirmed many of the things I was already doing in my family.

Barbara: My family avoided arguments at all costs, and I find that I am often paralysed and uncomfortable when couples become argumentative in sessions. I have had to work hard to find interventions to create a pause as my instinct is to be unsure about what is needed from me.

John: I was also thinking about the use of humour and that even out of serious events, we can find eternal hope. When I have experienced disruptions in my own life and relationships, I think it has helped me to use that knowledge sensitively with others and explore different possibilities that might emerge from problematic events.

Barbara: One personal story that endures with me is of some humiliating experiences in education which were critical and shaming. What I have chosen to take from them influences my activity with clients, supervisees, and students as I never use critical or shaming practices or language.

John: I remember you saying that you never criticise. I do, occasionally, but I hope I do it helpfully. It makes me think that any heartaches, doubts, separations in our lives could cast doubt on our professional abilities and we must work hard about taking feedback and knowing how to go on. I was thinking about my decision to change from practising as a structural therapist to the Milan approach. I thought the structural ideas did not reflect any of the families I had lived in and that the Milan approach opened up a more sympathetic view of families. Boscolo once said that it is not so important what the definition of the relationship is, but that the definition is clear. That has become a guiding principle in both personal and professional relationships.

John: Thinking about close relationships, I remember when I was 8, my Nana died. She was laid out in the bedroom that I shared with her. After the event I could not sleep, and my Mam asked if I was worried about ghosts. I said yes. Then she asked me: 'What kind of person had Nana been when she was alive?' I recalled lots of appreciative things and my Mam said, 'So what kind of ghost do you think she would be?' 'What kind of …..?' has become one of my best questions. I learned to play with language and frames of reference at a young age.

Barbara: This makes me think of the ways that we as professionals promote curiosity and freedom to find different ways of working.

> *John:* Yes, it is important to find a professional model that allows you to use the personal qualities that you have already got.
>
> *Barbara:* I always say to students, your theory will find you rather than you will find your theory because I think some ideas just land better with some people. At foundation level training, when professionals are encountering a range of ideas often for the first time, I invite students to 'think about the ideas that fit really well and learn to do them exceptionally well'.

Finding a Place for Feelings: Some Final Thoughts About Our Conversation

We are both drawn to notions of self, emotional and relational reflexivity as frames for exploring emotions in therapy and supervision (Burnham, 2005). We emphasize the exploration of transformational possibilities. Kolb (1984) suggests that we grasp the world from two different vantage points, one is concrete experience, which is our visceral response (sensing) and the other is abstract conceptualization which is about thinking (making sense).

> *Barbara:* As I name experiences in relation to turning points in my life, (paralyzed and uncomfortable or humiliating), I am less interested in the feelings themselves and more interested in using my concrete experience as a platform for reflective observation. This then enables me to work out how to think about the event and its utility in supervision thus creating the conditions for future active experimentation based on my newly achieved learning. In this way I can turn an emotionally reflexive moment into a relationally reflexive one. By doing so I am bringing an additional dimension to expressions of feelings from supervisees by encouraging them to be curious about their naming of emotions, the context within which they are likely to emerge and the effect on the work they do with others and any recalibration they may wish to make.
>
> *John:* In my early training I was coached **not** to ask about feelings, and to focus more on what people thought (about one another) and did (with each other). This early training has continued to influence me, though not as strongly as it once did. I am more likely to ask how people did/do *respond* to something. This allows the supervisee to begin where they

usually begin, and enables me to centre my inquiries wherever they start (meaning, feelings or action). In time I would connect and explore the relationship of their initial response to other aspects of their experience. For example. If someone begins with a thought, I can ask how they feel about that thought, and what does that feeling lead them to do and with whom. Feelings and emotions become part of a relational integration of experience.

References

Allen, K. (2012). What is an Ethical Dilemma? *The New Social Worker, 19*(2), xx–xx.

Burnham, J. (1992). Approach-method-technique: Creating distinctions and creating connections. *Human Systems, 3,* 3–27.

Burnham, J. (1993). Systemic supervision: The evolution of reflexivity in the context of the supervisory relationship. *Human Systems, 4*(3&4), 349–381.

Burnham, J. (2005). Relational reflexivity: A tool for socially constructing therapeutic relationships. In C. Flaskas, B. Mason, & A. Perlesz (Eds.), *The space between: Experience, context, and process in the therapeutic relationship.* Karnac Publications.

Burnham, J. (2012). Developments in social GRRRAAACCEEESSS: Visible-invisible and voiced-unvoiced. In I.-B. Kraus (Ed.), *Mutual perspectives: Culture and reflexivity in contemporary systemic psychotherapy.* Karnac Publications.

Burnham, J., & Nolte, L. (2020). 'Taking the plunge': How reflecting on your personal and social GgRRAAAACCEEEESSSS …..S can tame your restraints and refresh your resources. In J. Randall (Ed.), *Surviving clinical psychology: Navigating personal, professional and political selves on the journey to qualification.* Routledge.

Burnham, J., Twist, E., Brain, B., Maund, N., Desai, S., & Sigh, R. (2021). Manualising-personalising-without compromising (either the manual or the systemic approach) except when … In M. Mariotti, G. Saba, & P. Stratton (Eds.), *Handbook of systemic approaches to psychotherapy manuals: Integrating research, practice, and training.* Springer International (in press).

Cecchin, G. in conversation with Radovanovic, D. (1993). Prisoners of identity. *Human Systems, 4*, 3–18.

Clegg, J. (2004). How can services become more ethical? In W. R. Lindsay, J. L. Taylor, & P. Sturmey (Eds.), *Offenders with developmental disabilities*. Wiley.

Eisler, I. (2005). The empirical and theoretical base of family therapy and multiple family day therapy for adolescent anorexia nervosa. *Journal of Family Therapy, 27*, 104–131.

Freedman, J. & Combs, G. (1996). *Narrative therapy: The social construction of preferred realities*. Norton.

Karl, Cynthia, Andrew, & Vanessa. (1992). Therapeutic distinctions in an ongoing therapy. In S. McNamee & K. J. Gergen (Eds.), *Therapy as social construction*. Sage.

Kitchener, K. S., & Anderson, S. K. (2011). Thinking well about doing good. In K. S. Kitchener & S. K. Anderson (Eds.), *Foundations of ethical practice, research and teaching in psychology and counselling*. Routledge.

Kolb, D. (1984). *Experiential learning*. Prentice Hall.

McNamee, S. (2004). Promiscuity in the practice of family therapy. *Journal of Family Therapy, 26*(3), 224–244.

Pearce, W. B. & Cronen, V. E. (1980). *Communication, action and meaning*. Praeger.

Roper-Hall, A. (1998). Working systemically with older people and their families who have 'come to grief'. In P. Sutcliffe, G. Tufnell & U. Cornish (Eds.), *Working with the dying and bereaved: Systemic approaches to therapeutic work*. MacMillan Press.

Rorty, R. (1991). *Objectivity, relativism, and truth: Philosophical papers, Volume 1*. Cambridge University Press.

Skovholt, T. M., & Rønnestad, M. H. (1992). *The evolving professional self: Stages and themes in therapist and counsellor development*. Wiley and Sons.

Tomm, K. (1987). Interventive interviewing: Part II: Reflexive questioning as a means to enable self healing. *Family Process, 26*, 167–183.

Tomm, K. (1988). Interventive interviewing : Part III: Intending to ask lineal, circular, strategic or reflexive questions? *Family Process, 27*, 1–15.

Vetere, A., & Stratton, P. (2016). Interacting selves: Systemic solutions for personal and professional development in counselling and psychotherapy.

Watzlawick, P., Weakland, J., & Fisch, R. (1974). *Change: Principles of problem formation and problem resolution*. W.W. Norton & Company.

Wiener, N. (1953). The mutual influence of Physics and Medicine. Norbert Wiener Papers. MC 22 Box X Massachusetts. Massachusetts Institute of Technology, Institute Archives and Special Collections.

4

Relational Responsibility: Ethics and Power in Supervision

Sheila McNamee and Julie Tilsen

Introduction

It is clear that ethics cannot be formulated (Wittgenstein, 1961)

In this chapter, we outline and discuss ethics and issues of power in the relational process of supervision. Drawing on constructionist arguments, we introduce the shift from a sense of universal, stable ethics to a relational understanding of ethics which embraces respect for the potentially diverse constructions of what counts as ethical action present

---

S. McNamee (✉)
Department of Communication, University of New Hampshire, Durham, NH, USA
e-mail: sheila.mcnamee@unh.edu

J. Tilsen
2 Stories, Private Practice, Minneapolis, MN, USA
e-mail: julie@2stories.com

in the supervisory relationship. Power, following Foucault (1977), is similarly refigured as a description of interactive dynamics and not a quality of a person, thereby opening consideration of the supervisory relationship as not necessarily hierarchical. These revised understandings of ethics and power are aligned with the constructionist notion of relational responsibility (McNamee & Gergen, 1999). Unlike traditional notions of responsibility where individuals are held accountable for their actions, relational responsibility focuses on participants' attentiveness to processes of relating. This does not imply that people are not accountable for their actions but, contrary to our standard of individual responsibility where one's actions are viewed in isolation (on their own), relational responsibility reminds us that meaning is created in the joint actions and coordinations of all participants. In this sense, an ethic emerges as supervisor and supervisee engage with each other. No action is meaningful in itself. If supervisors, supervisees and clients are truly attentive to the process of relating, they extend possibilities for being relationally responsible.

Professional fields are fraught with a concern for ethical action where "ethical action" generally infers "doing the right thing" (referred to in this chapter as content ethics). In supervision, this translates into a reductive focus on ethics as a matter of minding institutional policies and obeying professional codes. Yet, when we operate within a relational sensibility—a world that embraces uncertainty as opposed to certainty, continual change as opposed to stability and local/historical/cultural contingencies rather than universal laws—answering the question, "what is ethical practice", requires an entirely different focus of attention.

In this chapter, we offer a pathway for clinical supervisors to make the shift from privileging institutional (content) ethics to centring relational processes in supervision. Doing so, we believe, supervisors invite clinicians to also centre relational processes in their direct service with clients.

Content or Process?

We introduce two forms of ethics: content ethics and process ethics. Content ethics refers to standards outlined in professional codes specifying how care givers should act in order to be accountable in their work with clients (e.g. confidentiality, issues of dual relationships, competence, etc.). In contrast, process ethics refers to the collaborative efforts and decisions of care givers and clients within each professional conversation. This can also be called conversational ethics, referring to the practical reasoning of supervisors and care givers and their situation-specific ways of conversing with clients/supervisees. One of the most important facets of a clinician's practice that supervisors are charged with fostering—and evaluating—is the ethicality of their practice.

Critical are invitations to supervisees to question supervisors' meanings and practices as a way of influencing and informing how the therapeutic and supervisory dialogue proceeds. Supervisor and supervisee negotiate their ways forward in the supervisory conversation. During this collaborative, negotiated dialogue, supervisors and supervisees are informed by how both content ethics and process ethics are transacted as they converse with clients.

This distinction between focus on content versus process is important. But it can also be misleading. We are not claiming that specific actions, deemed by communities, cultures or legal systems should be dismissed in favour of attention only to process. Rather, what we are saying is that first we should attempt to understand actions within the ongoing flow of—not only—the interactive moment but also within the ongoing flow of one's lived experiences and the meanings that have been constructed for those experiences. For example, abuse is wrong. Yet imprisoning an abuser does not guarantee reform. It does not transform those involved. But inquiring first into the lawbreaker's life narrative, into the trajectory that made the act of abuse "sensible", "a viable option" or "a required response" invites us into the constructed social order of the perpetrator. What is important here is the recognition that, from a constructionist stance, the perpetrator did not and does not construct his own social order; social orders emerge through the continued coordinations with others (see Figure 2.1 in Chapter 2). Thus, when we inquire into the perpetrator's life narrative, we enter into the co-constructed moral order that is relevant for him. We are genuinely curious about the micro-interactions with others that have generated a sense that a certain form of abuse is an appropriate response to a person, an action or a situation. The impulse to judge, evaluate and punish are held at bay while we first try to *understand* how such an action could be seen as reasonable *to the perpetrator*. When we enter into this space, the possibility of inviting this person into our more commonly shared (and legal) ethic is much greater. This does not mean sanctions will be abandoned. It does, however, mean that legal and cultural sanctions will be imposed in ways that have a greater chance to transform the wrongdoer.

We offer this radical approach with the understanding that accusations of guilt invite actions of self-defense. Schegloff and Sacks (1973) introduce us to the idea of adjacency pairs—the notion that the utterance or action of one person invites a particular response. These responses are cultivated over time, negotiated among people and eventually become automatic and anticipated responses. Examples include question/answer, invitation/acceptance and so on. Thus, in terms of ethics in supervision, we must recognize that our automatic, decontextualized accusation of guilt, wrong-doing or pathology will be responded to with some culturally normalized response and, that response, will most often be resistance. Approaching instead with curiosity and a genuine desire to understand (note: not agree or sanction) is likely to be met with an explanatory narrative.

Thus, how a supervisor approaches ethics (i.e. their view or the lens through which they view a therapist's practice) determines what kind of ethical stance they encourage in their supervisees. For example, consider the matter of multiple relationships (previously referred to as "dual relationships"). Imagine a high school student has been in therapy for a year. The student is about to graduate and invites her therapist to attend. The therapist seeks her supervisor's advice about the propriety of accepting the client's invitation to a personal, family event. If the supervisor is focused on content ethics, adherence to one-size-fits-all agency policies that prohibit engaging in non-professional activities and maintaining a strictly professional relationship would guide the supervisor's advice. There is no consideration of the possible beneficial therapeutic impact of a therapist attending the graduation; rather, the personal nature of the invitation restricts the supervisor's acceptance (Tilsen, 2021). Conversely, a supervisor who is adhering to the notion of relational responsibility would consider an array of contextual, cultural, and circumstantial factors that centre the client's worldview and needs, while also considering the demands and expectations of his/her professional context. These considerations might include, for example, the client's cultural norms, matters of confidentiality and privacy, considering the harm done to the client by *not doing* what may be prohibited by professional codes or agency policies, the meaning a client makes of the therapist's action and the potential impact on others involved.

Questioning the Tradition: From Stability to Fluidity of Ethics

Our thinking about ethics traditionally has been issue or action based. By this we mean that we judge actions—typically isolated from the contexts in which they emerge—as ethical or unethical. This means that we ignore the flow of ongoing interaction. Attending a client's event, touching a client, giving a client a ride, accepting a gift from a client and seeing a client with whom you have a prior connection—all are deemed as questionable actions by many state licensing boards and agencies. Within the tradition of ethics, all actions can (or should) be determined as right or wrong, good or bad. In this chapter, we certainly do not intend to argue that abuse, incest, crime or violence are acceptable actions. At the same time, we raise for consideration those licensing boards that would see acceptance of a gift from a client as unethical action. While the space between accepting a gift and incest, crime or violence is vast, we raise these extremes in an attempt to call attention to the ways in which a code of ethics can—at both extremes—impact the lives of clients and therapists, supervisors and supervisees. Once we step into a relational orientation where we acknowledge right and wrong, good and bad as meanings crafted in community with others—always situated within historical, cultural and local contexts—what we claim as our ethical actions, themselves, can be questioned—particularly by the standards of some other meaning-making community. In other words, we need to be thoughtful and reflexive before assuming what is and is not ethical action so the above actions, such as accepting a gift from a client or giving them a lift home, cannot simply be judged as unethical or ethical by a set of professional codes. We privilege the relational context and the relational process over a detached assessment of an action.

To be sure, more or less stable communities, families and traditions can confidently claim right and wrong within a specific context, but step outside that community, that family or that tradition and what is deemed good may likely appear evil, wrong or immoral. This is because what we come to view as ethical and just action is worked out in the relational coordination of people in interaction (Bava & McNamee, 2019).

The Danger of Being Seduced by Traditional Ethics: Power and Authority

Let us address the dangers of resorting to a traditional sense of ethics. In particular, we would like to address the possible harm we commit when supervisors let practice be guided solely by the professional code of ethics. But first, we should be clear: we are not calling for a total abandonment of any code of ethics by which we pledge to practise. We are simply hoping to raise awareness that, while created with the best of intentions (to protect those clients with whom we work, as well as ourselves and the agencies or institutions within which we work), the unilateral and decontextualized use of pre-determined ethical codes can be, themselves, unethical and destructive.

Like any other generalized knowledge, ethics arise out of agreements achieved by a group of highly trained professionals. What becomes the ethical cannon in the area of social care is reached through a slow and arduous process where cases are presented and examined, opinions are shared, and evidence—in the form of scientific research—is reviewed. While we might prefer to believe that it is not the case, we would be remiss to ignore that, during deliberation, those with more authority and power and/or those with exceptional verbal abilities will dominate the discussion thereby encouraging (often experienced more as forcing) others to agree with a preferred analysis leading to a specific ethical practice. This raises the issue of power and authority as they enter into our attempts to coordinate multiple worldviews as we, in this one specific illustration, attempt to develop agreement upon a code of ethics. Additionally, we question if unanimity of opinion is even possible or desirable? This question challenges us to consider replacing the value of unanimity with the coordination of difference. However, both power and unanimity need further discussion.

Power as an Obstruction to Coordinating Multiplicity. We are all familiar with consensus-as-agreement emerging out of the silencing of some voices. We have all been part of groups where the attempt to "do the right thing" is assumed to be achievable via democratic vote. Let us say, in an attempt to expand your services within the community, a special meeting is called for all staff of your organization. The question is posed: Should there be a weekend retreat to discuss how to expand services? This option would allow uninterrupted work during the week. Or should there be a series of weekly meetings allowing staff and colleagues personal time on their weekends? A vote is taken. Let's imagine that the majority of the staff members are senior (i.e. older) with little to no family responsibilities, given their life stage, while the minority have young children and family obligations. In this case, it is not only "those with family obligations" pitted against "those without family obligations", but it is "younger – perhaps less-secure-staff" against "senior staff". When the vote is called, the senior staff members are quick to voice their preference for one weekend retreat—"a good opportunity to hash out this issue!" The younger staff members, feeling dependent on remaining in the good graces of their senior colleagues, feel obligated to go along with the majority. Thus, the so-called democratic choice is a weekend retreat.

Has this group coordinated their differences? We do not think any of us would say that they have. Rather, the powerful voice of the majority has silenced alternative voices. Instead of promoting a coordination of diverse perspectives and a collaborative process, the opposite occurs: relationships fraught with submerged antagonisms are created and division is ignited.

What if this were the way in which ethical principles were developed? Do we have any reason to assume that the deliberation concerning what comes to count as a professional's ethical behaviour would transpire in any other way? While the very points we raise here have actually been taken into consideration as the professional community debated two contemporary "hot" issues—the DSM-5 (Dillon, 2013; Reardon, 2014) and Evidence-Based Practice (Milton, 2005)—there is little (or no) concern for examining how ethical codes emerge through group (committee) processes of construction.

Unanimity as an Obstruction to Coordinating Multiplicity. Our lives are populated with anything but unanimity. We are bombarded by diverse and competing viewpoints and belief systems daily—even by our closest companions. We see the clash of opposing traditions everywhere. In a world of diversity, is it desirable to valorize unanimous opinion, as if we were all "of one mind?" What might be lost when we set for ourselves the goal of consensus-as-agreement? Whose voices are silenced in the name of unanimity and at what superficial level are our agreements solidified?

Consensus of this sort minimizes difference, erasing the very struggles that generate a dynamic and diverse public sphere. With so many traditions, beliefs and values to coordinate, how could unanimity be possible? The world is complex, not simple. It is time that we develop ways of coordinating complexity rather than eliminating it. After all, wouldn't it be more generative to replace the impulse to agree (or to medicate) with the impulse to be curious about differences? Let's not define coordination of difference as agreement; let's define it as understanding (where understanding does not mean agreement, evaluation or judgement—it simply means generating curiosity about difference). Our respectful attempts to understand might foster new forms of collaborative activity and this collaboration might enhance tolerance of difference. We might find that a person who appears depressed is facing daunting issues of unemployment, poor health and financial debt. Another one who appears paranoid, upon further discussion, tells of his family's attempt to make sure he is never alone (after convincing him that they are not worried about his well-being). Furthermore, such understanding might pave the

4 Relational Responsibility: Ethics and Power in Supervision

way for a relationally sensitive ethic, one that is attuned to culture, tradition, specific relations and the very local context within which certain ways of being have transpired.

Consider public discussion focused on resolving the issue of diagnosis and medication. We know already that there are diverse views on this topic. Yet, consider this: no one is born with a position for or against the issue. Rather, the positions we adopt are worked out in the give and take of our conversations with others—family, friends, acquaintances, religious communities, professional enclaves and media. The position we take on this issue emerges from interactions that are most central to us. And, while discussing this topic with others who share the same opinion, we experience a particular form of coordinated action that confirms and substantiates our view—we feel certain and righteous.

Reflect for a moment on the various issues about which you are passionate. Think about some of your strongest beliefs. Over what issue or issues would others claim you lose your "objectivity?" What are the topics you have a difficult time discussing with others? Now think about the conversations, the interactions and the relational histories where you feel supported and virtuous for your stance on these heated issues.

It is rare that we enter into interaction with others curious of their coherence (like the murderer, the sexual assaulter or the combative partner)—if they disagree with us (professionals), they are wrong. We rarely ask for detailed descriptions of how and why their very different view has emerged as viable and logical and for whom. Instead, we typically enter into these interactions with the idea of persuading others to accept our view as the "right" view. And yet, if we enter into supervision with the hope of understanding differences rather than attempting to reach agreement (i.e. persuade), we are more likely to forge new relational and interactional possibilities. We are much more likely to stay in conversation with someone who genuinely wants to understand our position than with one who simply attacks or claims we are wrong. Note how abandoning the desire for consensus-as-agreement opens us to the possibility of creating new forms of understanding with others. We are no longer talking about universal good or bad, right or wrong but good and bad, right or wrong that are worked out at a very local level. This is the shift from "consensus-as-agreement" to processes of engagement that build understanding of diversity and, thereby create community—common ground. Can we dissolve the dichotomy of incommensurate worldviews by creating opportunities where we can engage in interested inquiry and curiosity with others? And, in dissolving the good/bad, right/wrong dichotomies we encounter in supervisory conversations, can we achieve some form of coordinated social action where diversity is initially approached with tolerance and respect? Can we imagine—and more important, can we create—a social order that is not ordered by similarity but is ordered by coordination of diversity? To do so embodies a relational ethic.

Thinking about relational ethics as an ethic of "discursive potential" (McNamee, 2015) helps us focus on working towards understanding first, rather than judgement. Maintaining a focus on creating opportunities for understanding in supervision underscores the everyday co-construction of ethics between supervisor and supervisee.

To that end, relational supervision centres our attention on both the collaborative nature of any interaction as well as the responsivity of all participants to each other and the environment/context. Bakhtin (1981) claims that our words and actions are not entirely our own; they carry our history of relationships and the beliefs and values these relationships have crafted. This is a foundational concept in social construction: the words we use carry meanings shaped by multiple others, and people hear our words and make meaning of them based on their experiences, also shaped by multiple others. This responsivity—this recognition—of the many relations our words and actions carry is possible within a relational ethic where attentiveness to the process of relating is centred (process ethics), rather than adherence to some abstract, decontextualized set of principles (content ethics). A relationally sensitive practice respects the diversity of locally situated beliefs and values, as discussed in prior chapters. Responsivity allows practitioners to let go of imposing judgement, assessment and evaluation of others' actions and opens the door for attentiveness to the coordination of diverse social orders. This marks a significant departure from the tradition of supervision—or the common cultural understanding of it—where it is assumed that evaluation, correction or guidance are central.

For example, a supervisor might ask a supervisee questions about his or her intentions or about the actual effects of their practice on clients. What the clients might say in response to the clinician's comments, suggestions or questions could also be an illustration of attending to how supervisor and supervisee attempt to coordinate multiple perspectives. Such a stance departs from the directive approach of traditional supervision where the supervisor knows best and imparts his/her wisdom and advice on the supervisee. Instead, a relationally reflexive (Burnham, 2005) conversation between supervisor and supervisee allows for a conversation about how one positions oneself, how one's practice invites or closes down possibilities. It allows for an acknowledgement of our part in constructing the unfolding process.

Self-Reflexivity

From a relational stance, our responsivity to others—particularly to others who seek our "expert" opinion—opens us to examining our own commitments and beliefs. Such an examination—known as self-reflexivity—is critical to a constructionist stance. Self-reflexivity takes the form of inner dialogue where we question our own certainty, entertain alternative understandings and imagine what meaning others might attribute to the present situation.

In the supervisory context, self-reflexivity assists us in avoiding the adoption of the expert stance and instead invites us into that collaborative moment of co-construction. The impulse to offer advice is replaced with the invitation to think together about alternative interpretations and alternative forms of action. It takes the form of inner dialogue where we ask ourselves, "Would this be a useful way to approach this case?" "How might others approach this?" "Am I being curious enough?" Such questions open space and facilitate the ongoing supervisory conversation. They also invite the supervisee into a fully participatory scenario rather than an evaluative or instructive one. Adopting a self reflexive stance allows supervisors to engage in curious inquiry about their own practice of supervision. Such curious inquiry often becomes the source of new questions for the supervisee that, in turn, invite the supervisee into a reflexive stance vis a vis his/her own practice.

Attention to how one's questions, comments and observations invite or delimit possibilities is critical. There are no neutral observations, questions or comments. And, at the same time, we are not suggesting that supervisors continually struggle to find the "right" comments or observations. Rather, what we are proposing is that supervisors, like supervisees, continually monitor how their actions (comments, questions, observations, suggestions) invite particular responses. And, if undesired responses emerge, the supervisor (just as the supervisee with his/her client) can offer an alternative which might shift the response and facilitate a way forward.

Reflexivity offers a way of being responsive as opposed to reactive. It requires questioning one's own world view just enough to allow space for the rationality of the other's view. The focus is on making space for multiple rationalities. In professional practice, this means that our job is not to impose our "expert" understanding on the other but to create a space where multiple (and often diverse) understandings can co-exist. Within a relational ethic we are less focused on what we are doing and saying and are more attentive to the processes in which we are engaged and how our actions invite each other into particular patterns and relationships; we are focused on the ever-unfolding nature of meaning.

Cultivating Reflexivity: From Private to Public

How can we make alternative understandings visible to clients? We suggest a process of *reflection, deconstruction and curiosity*. As a practice activity, we can consider various clinical scenarios and pose the following questions. The questions centre on developing one's reflexivity (entertaining doubt about certainties), considering multiple perspectives and interrogating power/normativity.

For example, consider the following situation:

You work at a clinic that serves a large number of LGBT clients. Your client, a 45-year-old white cisgender man, is adamant that he is "going to hell" for his "uncontrollable desires" of being attracted to men. He does not identify as gay, bi, or queer; he refers to "homosexual acts" when speaking about his desires and sexual activities. He keeps asking you to perform conversion therapy. He's clear about liking you and feeling comfortable with you; it's just that he wants you to "fix" him. You keep seeing him, but you are strongly opposed to conversion therapy, which you tell him every time he asks about it. To top it off, you're queer, and he knows this.

First, consider these questions for **reflection**:

- What are your initial reactions and thoughts about this?
- What might be a stance identified as content ethics?
- What about this stance is important to you and why?

Next, **deconstruct** your understanding:

- What are the assumptions and values that your initial reactions are based on and what do those assumptions and values reflect?
- Whose assumptions and values are privileged (what discourses, institutions, influences, etc. do they represent) within the stance of conventional ethics?
- What actions or decisions might this stance lead you to? What might the effects be? On whom?

And finally, adopt a **curiosity** about the vignette presented:

- What considerations might you entertain from a stance of process ethics (relational responsibility)?
- What or whose other perspectives could you take?
- What might these perspectives make possible?
- What are some specific questions you could ask about this stance?

By applying this process of reflection, deconstruction and curiosity to situations that are particular to your own context, you will cultivate your capacity for reflexivity and open space for a proliferation of understandings and ways of being in the world. This fosters a relational ethic that is responsive, accountable and positions us in collaboration with those who consult us.

Relational Responsibility

Ethics, within a constructionist stance, embraces a very particular understanding of responsibility. It is, as discussed earlier, a relational responsibility (McNamee & Gergen, 1999) or, simply, it is attentiveness to the process of relating, itself. We no longer concern ourselves with individual responsibility because to do so would position supervisor, supervisee and client as decontextualized ethical agents. Relational responsibility is in contrast to conventional professional (content) ethics in which there is often little to no regard for the very local, historical and situational contingencies of the interactive moment. From the stance of content ethics, actions are deemed responsible and ethical if they meet some abstract professional standard.

Furthermore, it's critical to name that content ethics come from, reflect and perpetuate white, patriarchal norms (Tilsen, 2021). These norms reproduce patriarchal hierarchies of knowledge (whose knowledge counts and whose does not) and thus further marginalize the already most marginalized. Content ethics is a product of the medical model and the positivist tradition and, as such, reflects the assumptions of client pathology and professional expertise inherent within these approaches. Greenspan (1995) calls this approach to ethics and practice the "distance model". In the distance model, professional expertise is privileged over client knowledge, and relational mutuality is seen as harmful to therapeutic outcome (Dietz & Thompson, 2004). Viewed through a Foucauldian lens, we see content ethics as maintaining disciplinary power (Foucault, 1977); content ethics serve as surveillance over clinical practice.

We note that when organizations and professions attend to relational processes, as argued here, there will be a sensitivity to ongoing and unfolding practices that will invite adjusting, rewriting and instituting new policies otherwise known as content ethics. For example, attention to particular forms of language use or discriminatory practices may well be introduced into the content ethic canon. Yet, despite the good intentions of revising an organization's or profession's content ethics, they remain static and can, therefore, be employed in harmful ways such as policing a clinician's language use with a client when, in fact, that language has been mutually agreed upon. In contrast, process ethics are, by definition, dynamic (i.e. responsive, fluid and emergent). We acknowledge the problem of using the binary of content/process and suggest that process always includes content—it is always in relation to content. To that end, any formal ethical code would require constant revision due to the evolving nature of human interaction. And, if a profession's or organization's ethical code was continually being revised, any "violation" would require (demand in fact) inquiry into the interactive moment, the situated activity and the multiplicity of meanings emerging rather than the typical by-product of content ethics which is the levelling of sanctions.

In supervision, the distance model leads supervisors to conflate ethics with legality and centre professional/agency priorities as opposed to those that reflect the values and needs of therapists and the people with whom they work. For example, a school-based therapist working with children under 12 years old was told by her supervisor to avoid all "physical contact" including "side" hugs and handshakes with the children. "Highfives" were the only kind of touch approved, regardless of the situation. This was in response to the district's legal department issuing a statement about not touching children and clearly ignored any consideration of the values and needs of the children (or the therapist).

Can we honestly call such decontextualized activities responsible or ethical? Social construction, with its relational focus, presents a challenge to traditional notions of expert knowledge and professional neutrality, as we have already discussed. It is not the case that constructionists do not recognize expertise or authority. What constructionists challenge is the unquestioned presumption that the professional should be the authority (and that it is only in the professional's position as authority or expert that success can be accomplished). We would like to suggest that the task at hand is one of coordination among professional, client and the broader community within which they operate. Such coordination requires abandoning any pre-determined understanding and being open to explore the social orders of those with whom we work. That coordination might include problem talk, diagnosis and an authoritative stance taken by the professional. It is also likely that it might require the professional to adopt the stance of an equal conversational partner who does not know with certainty how to understand or make sense of the client's problem. Furthermore, it might involve conversation about possibilities, potentials and ideals. The point is, from a constructionist stance, we cannot know ahead of time what will be most generative for any professional/client relationship.

The uncertainty that is associated with a constructionist stance is one that invites multiplicity and thereby invites supervisors and supervisees alike to question their assumptions and explore alternative resources for personal, relational and social transformation—this is the reflexive space that Burnham and McKay discuss in Chapter 3. We could call this uncertainty "generative uncertainty", a term that we believe echoes Wittgenstein's (1961) notion about a decontextualized ethic, "It is clear that ethics cannot be formulated". Generative uncertainty positions supervisor and supervisee in a relationship that is responsive to the interactive moment. The supervisor is now a conversational partner and as such is free to move within the relationship in ways that enhance both supervisor's and supervisee's abilities to draw on a wide range of conversational resources.

The supervisor is not burdened with being "right" but with being present and responsive. The supervisor and supervisee become accountable to each other. Yet, accountability, presence and responsivity to each other is not enough. Our conversations might be more usefully centred on community transformation. How might we invite clients into the sorts of relationships that effectively transform our ways of living communally? To that end, relational supervision would suggest that clinical ethics expand well beyond the supervisor/supervisee relationship. One way to embrace the stance of relational responsibility is to understand our questions as inviting ethical positionings.

Ethics as Questions. Instead of thinking about ethical questions, we make a shift to ethics as questions (Freedman & Combs, 1996). Ethics as questions facilitates the shift from rules to relationships, as we engage not with stagnant codes of conduct, but a generative inquiry process centred on our relationships with people, our work, our values and the effects of what we do on these relationships.

Intentionally and critically questioning what we do and what our doing creates (Foucault, 1977), fosters accountability for our practice.

This is an accountability *to* those we work with, not an accountability *for* them. This is an important shift, one which rejects the implicit (if not explicit) paternalism embedded within conventional professional ethics (Professional Knows Best) and replaces it with attention to the power relations inherent in therapist-client and supervisor-worker relationships.

There are three practice domains within which we focus this inquiry. These areas include: the examination of practices (questions about the values and relationships your practice brings forward); examination of power (questions about people, relationships and whose voice prevails); and examination of the effects of practice (questions for evaluating your practice which are based on the effects of your practice on people, not on rule compliance).

Here we propose some generative questions based on these three areas of examination:

- How does this model or theory view people?
- How does it expect you to show up and act in your work and particularly in relationship with clients/supervisees?
- How does it expect clients/supervisees to view you and act with you?
- How would you describe the positioning encouraged by this practice?
- Who is considered to have knowledge and expertise?
- Who enters whose world?
- Does this way of doing therapy foster normativity or generativity? How?
- What are the effects of this practice on people, on their relationships with important other people in their lives, and on the communities to which they belong?
- What is valued in this model or theory? What is devalued or disvalued? (adapted from Freedman and Combs, 1996).

Everyday Ethics

The topic of ethics has become somewhat of an appendage to practise, something that we consider in the context of risk management, dilemmas and legal matters. We contend that "ethics is the blood that courses through the body of our practice" (Tilsen, 2018, p. 37) and as such, is a matter of everyday practice.

Addressing these everyday matters in supervision means we help supervisees engage in critically questioning the normative assumptions ungirding these taken-for-granted clinical practices. These assumptions are located in both our professional and dominating cultural contexts and reflect normative ideas about race, class, gender, sexuality, ability, culture, age, etc. Below are some "everyday" clinical situations that we think merit a more thorough consideration of whose ethics are centred, the practices that emerge from those centred ethics, and what the effects of those practices are:

- Meeting w/individual for a relational issue
- Seeing a child w/o the parents
- Diagnosis & the privatization of social problems
- "Anger management" in an unjust world, used as a tool of social control
- Supervision/consultation without client
- "Managing" behaviour; Notions of "normal" perpetuating prevailing, specifying, and oppressive discourses and systems of power
- Continuing services w/o change or improvement.

Addressing these issues also means that, as supervisors, we help supervisees cultivate and articulate their own intentions and aspirations for their relational ethics. Reynolds (2014) advocates for a practice of centring ethics, in which we make visible our ethical framework. Thus, unlike conventional therapy practice and supervision in which we organize our work around treatment goals or performance of specific models or techniques, we organize our work around our ethics and the effects of what we do. Centring ethics helps us embody our values and cultivate practices of accountability by making our ethics public.

What does this look like in practice? Supervisors can ask therapists how they make real their stated intentions of, for example, practising in anti-oppressive ways, doing social justice work, and being culturally responsive (Reynolds, 2014). One team I (Julie) provided clinical supervision for had positioned itself in the community to work with families who have queer and transgender youth. As we talked together about their shared ethic of "being accessible and responsive to all families", we talked about what this meant and how they would hold themselves to this. I asked questions not only about their direct practices with families, but also about their agency's leadership, policies, written materials, staffing, etc. This led to team members initiating an agency-wide revamping of policies and procedures (from hiring practices, to clinical training, to paperwork and EHR language, to client involvement in policy and programme decisions) in order for them to be able to demonstrate that they were practising in alignment with their stated ethics.

Assuming that therapists are therapists because they want to make a difference that their clients value, we can also assume that they want to practise in ways that support this intention. In our experience as supervisors, often when practitioners feel stuck and frustrated, when they complain of "burn out", or view clients as "resistant", it is because they are practising in ways that inhibit their ability to live into their ethics (Reynolds, 2011). It is no surprise that this happens since clinical training more and more emphasizes fidelity to treatment approaches not to clients, and ethics is presented in a reductive and detached-from-daily practice manner. Most forms of supervision follow suit and focus on models and techniques, keeping the ethical framework hidden until dilemmas are addressed. Relational supervision attends to helping clinicians acknowledge, interrogate and learn how to practise and make visible their commitment to relationally responsible therapeutic processes.

We also assume supervisors supervise because they want to help therapists cultivate their practice. They want to help therapists make a difference in people's lives by practising in ways that are both meaningful and sustainable. Supervisors who approach ethics from a stance of relational responsibility invite therapists into conversational spaces that centre client knowledges, emphasize partnership, consider context and power relations and expand ethics to encompass all relational engagement. We believe that supervisors who centre ethics in this way provide therapists with a supportive and generative alternative to the distant and institutional ethics typically practised.

References

Bakhtin, M. M. (1981). *The dialogic imagination: Four essays* (M. Holquist, Ed.; C. Emerson & M. Holquist, Trans.). University of Texas Press.

Bava, S., & McNamee, S. (2019). Imagining relationally crafted justice: A pluralist stance. *Contemporary Justice Review, 22*(3), 290–306.

Burnham, J. (2005). Relational reflexivity: A tool for socially constructing therapeutic relationships. In C. Flaskas, B. Mason, & A. Perlesz (Eds.), *The space between: Experience, context, and process in the therapeutic relationship* (pp. 1–18).

Dietz, C., & Thompson, J. (2004). Rethinking boundaries: Ethical dilemmas in the social worker-client relationship. *Journal of Progressive Human Services, 15*(2), 1–24.

Dillon, J. (2013). Hearing voices network launches debate on DSM-5 and psychiatric diagnosis. http://www.madinamerica.com/2013/05/hearing-voices-network-launches-debate-on-dsm-5-and-psychiatric-diagnoses/. Retrieved 24 January 2015.

Foucault, M. (1977). *Discipline and punish: The birth of the prison* (A. Sheridan, Trans.). Vintage Books.

Freedman, J. & Combs, G. (1996). *Narrative therapy: The social construction of preferred realities*. W. W. Norton.

Greenspan, M. (1995, July/August). Out of bounds. In *Common boundary* (pp. 51–58).

McNamee, S. (2015). Ethics as discursive potential. *The Australian and New Zealand Journal of Family Therapy, 36*, 419–433.

McNamee, S., & Gergen, K. J. (1999). *Relational responsibility: Resources for sustainable dialogue*. Sage.

Milton, M. (2005). The ethics (or not) of evidence-based practice. In R. Tribe, & J. Morrissey (Eds.), *Handbook of professional and ethical practice for psychologists, counsellors and psychotherapists*. Brunner-Routledge.

Reardon, C. (2014). DSM-5—Debate, soul searching, changes. *Social Work Today, 14*(3), 10.

Reynolds, V. (2011). Resisting burnout with justice-doing. *International Journal of Narrative Therapy and Community Work, 4*, 27–45.

Reynolds, V. (2014). Centering ethics in group supervision: Fostering cultures of critique and structuring safety. *International Journal of Narrative Therapy and Community Work, 1*, 1–13.

Schegloff, E. A., & Sacks, H. (1973). Opening up closings. *Semiotica, 7,* 289–327.

Tilsen, J. (2018). *Narrative approaches to youthwork: Conversational skills for a critical practice.* Routledge.

Tilsen, J. (2021). *Queering your therapy practice: Queer theory, narrative therapy, and imagining new identities.* Routledge.

Wittgenstein, L. (1961). *Tractatus logico-philosophicus.* Routledge.

5

Making the Combination of Support and Social Control Work in Supervision

Øyvind Kvello

Introduction

The focus of this chapter is supervising professionals who have double mandates because they combine help and social control. The Norwegian Child Protection Service (CPS) operates with such a two-part mandate as described, but the issue is transferable to several professions and businesses. The double mandate can be ethically and professionally challenging: After some time where professionals are helping the family, the children are moved to an institution or in foster care due to lack of good enough care. This is often experienced by the families as betrayals. Information that professionals helping families accomplishes can be held against the parents and used as information for the court, where they

---

Ø. Kvello (✉)
Department of Education and Lifelong Learning, Norwegian University of Science and Technology, Trondheim, Norway
e-mail: oyvind.kvello@ntnu.no

decide if children should live in foster care or institutions for a long time, or adoption of the child.

Central themes that emerge in supervision of professionals at CPS are: Handling resistance by being transparent, supporting the development of intrinsic motivation (may be developed by the use of externalizing the problem and Motivational Interviewing), and creating strong and often long-lasting working alliances. The mentalization-based and attachment-strengthening intervention Circle of Security uses the metaphors of "the circle of care" for the tasks that caregivers have, and "hands" for caregivers' support when children are exploring and "hands" when children need support. Supervisors often are the "hands" that holds the professionals when they feel being on the top of the circle and have a sense of mastery, as well as offering comforting when they feel like being on the bottom of the circle. In the same way, professionals should be the hands for parents, and parents should be supported to be the hands for their children.

The Core Dimensions of Supervision

Supervising social workers at CPS in England is assumed to cover several needs (Manthorpe et al., 2013): (1) contributing to the use of research-based knowledge, (2) guarding against burnout and (3) work satisfaction and reductions in turnover. Many professionals, inside as well as outside, are encouraged to use supervisors, as they perceive supervision as an important contribution for ensuring professionals to held high-quality standards. The concept of supervision often includes three themes: (1) discussing clients of CPS to gain the social worker's understanding of families. This should primarily be based on empirical and theoretical knowledge. (2) Developing practical competence, i.e. transforming empirical and theoretical knowledge into a know-how by the social workers. (3) Reflections on being a social worker, which includes: professional identity, personal strengths and weaknesses, reflections on job content and understanding CPS as an organization.

These three themes are tied together with relational processes, and the supervisors forming trustful relationships with the professionals supervised. To be supervised involves being vulnerable by presenting shortcomings and doubts, for example, concerns about cases that are not progressing or turns out as well as expected and how this impact on the professional's sense of professional competency and growth.

The Metaphors of Adding Versus Redeeming

As described, there are three broad themes included in supervision, but what is included in the role of or expectations professionals held for supervisors? Supervisors might portray themselves as responsible for adding knowledge to the social workers. Supervisors are often experienced and therefore share their knowledge during supervisions. The metaphor of adding knowledge is based on the assumptions of supervisor as an expert. Supervision based on sharing knowledge can lead to dependency, i.e. it would take a long time for workers at CPS to develop a similar competence as very experienced supervisors possesses, partly because CPS is a broad and complex field, and the turnover is often high. But sharing knowledge can sometimes lead to supervisees' growth as professionals when setting their own goals, and not primarily trying to compete with the supervisor.

The metaphor of redeeming is an opposite to the metaphor of adding. Redeeming is rooted on empowering the social worker. The role of the supervisor is perceived as a catalyst that encourages the social workers to use their knowledge. The supervisors are restraint of adding their knowledge. Instead, they will encourage the social workers to build on their own experiences and knowledge. Supervision based on redeeming is a parallel to empowerment.

Words Are Not Neutral or Innocent

According to Andersen (1996), words are not passive of emotionally neutral. Words are touching and moving. Talking are informing and forming. The way supervisors talk about clients and ethical dilemmas influence the values and attitudes of the social workers. In a way, this could be described as hidden learning processes of influence, as the process is based on model learning—and the social workers imitating the supervisor.

Suggestions for the Social Worker–Supervisor Relationship

The conscious use of words is not just seen in formulations of questions and what kind of information they can give, but also the labels the supervisors use in order to describe and sum up the information. Supervision is often about working on two levels: (1) on a concrete level: offering interpretations regarding cases presented and giving advices, (2) as well as an abstract level: the supervisors ask circular, reflexive and relational questions as well as commenting on the ongoing process (using a meta-language). Supervisors have a marked influence when responding to and re-framing of words and expressions from the social workers in supervisions. Supervisors should be aware of adding nuances to what is told and highlight parts of great importance. The effect of supervisors' summaries is often influential.

Supervising on How to Handle Family Resistance

There are at least five obvious reasons for families to develop resistance towards CPS: (1) They often disagree with parts of or all of the referral, (2) CPS have a bad reputation among many peoples, (3) it is difficult for some families to relate to the combination of help and control given from the CPS, (4) there is an imbalance of power between the families and the workers at CPS and (5) as professionals the perspectives and definitions by the CPS often weigh heavier than the opinions that families have.

An Explanation for the Referral

For some families, it can be useful to talk with the person(s) that wrote the referral to CPS. The persons who made the referral can explain their concern for the children and why they find it necessary to ask on the behalf of the family for help from CPS. Sometimes the persons behind the referrals to the CPS are private and sometimes anonymous. According to Norwegian law, CPS cannot ask private persons to meet the family for explaining the motivation for referral. For referrals made by professionals, one can ask them to meet the family for a conversation. Professionals can refuse to meet the family, but mine and others' experience are that some want to meet the family. Professionals that send referrals sometimes inform and explain for the family why they send the referral and the content. In these situations, families often do not feel a need for talking with the professionals, but when referral is sent without informing the family about it.

The Imbalance of Power

As often in counselling and therapy, there is an imbalance of intimate sharing because the social worker at CPS often learns the client's deepest secrets while the client usually knows only superficial facts about the social worker. This can create a vulnerability as well as imbalance of power (Lazarus et al., 2019).

Three out of four families referred to the Norwegian CPS belong to the two lowest out of nine socio-economical levels (Martinsen & Lichtwarck, 2013), while social workers belong to lower middle class. In addition, most social workers are white, while a great amount of client of CPS have immigrant background.[1]

If the situations for the child are defined by the CPS as severe, the family cannot "fire" the social worker. It can even be difficult for families to ask for another social worker when feeling they do not achieve a trustful relationship, due to logistic and capacity or if the wish for

---

[1] Statistics of Norway (2019) report that 18.2% of the Norwegian population are immigrants or born in Norway with immigrant parents.

a change of social worker is understood as manipulative behaviour or attempts to split the employees in two diametrically opposed groups.

Suggestions for the Social Worker–Supervisor Relationship

These issues presented above can create an imbalance of power that can amplify the resistance towards the CPS. Common to these obstacles described are that the imbalance cannot be solved, e.g. the socio-economical differences, ethnicity, gender and problems to change social worker if the families are not satisfied with the professionals they got. Supervisors should on regular basis highlight these perspectives and encourage the social workers to discuss these with the family. Even though these issues cannot be solved, it can be helpful for the families to reflect upon them and to experience that the social worker to be preoccupied by them and not trivialize the imbalance of power. Being humble in relation to these issues is a respectful way of being in relation to families.

Coping with Conflicting Discourses

The best way to reduce resistance and scepticism against CPS is probably by supervisors that encourages the social workers to be a transparent as possible and to have no hidden agendas.[2] Supervisors can enhance such practice by using a meta-language where they talk about the reflections and motives for the advices given as well as commenting in this way when the social workers reflect upon how to understand and help the family. In this way, supervisors can facilitate reflections of how they act and their true feelings and opinions.

---

[2]There is an exception to the rule when the professionals suspect that the child is exposed to family violence, sexual or physical abuse, to avoid misuse of evidence.

Listening to the Voices of the Families

Some families express their despair of not being listened to by the CPS. They feel their perspective do not count and that the perspectives held by the social workers are completely dominating (Martinsen & Lichtwarck, 2013). The law is clear when it comes to who is responsible for the professionally based assessments, but this can be done in a very authoritarian way or in an inviting style. The wording inviting style does not mean to let the families do the assessments but let their voices to be heard. It works well to site their reflections and involve them during the assessment. For example, when mapping risk and protective factors, the social worker can write down their opinions, but at the same time also write down the opinions for each family member. Supervisors can encourage the social workers to discuss similarities and differences in opinion between family members as well as the family versus the social worker. A curious exploration is not just letting the family voices to be heard but can be a fruitful way for the social worker to understand each of the family members.

The majority of those who refer families to CPS are professionals, members of the social network or neighbours that want professional help for the family or is worried for the parents' care for the children. The family often disagrees with the expressed concern in the referral, for the families are often surprised by the referral and feel hurt by the content of it. They often express ambivalence or disagreement, but some of the families report some relief because the help they will receive. The family's perspectives should be heard and documented in the journal, for it should be possible for them to counter the information given in the referral. Supervisors can establish or enhance this practice by asking for the families' perspectives and how the social worker deal with them and document them.

Assessing Challenges and Resources

Some families report that CPS are looking for difficulties and describes this in detail. It goes at the expense of assessing the resources and strengths. The law requires that challenges are assessed in order to decide whether the care of the child is good enough, but in order to understand the family in nuanced ways, the strengths of the family ought to be discovered and included as a part of the assessment. Resources are important to build on when helping the family to increased quality of life and to strengthen parents caring skills.

To Confirm Intense Feelings

The families' reactions on the referral, the imbalance of power between them and the social worker can be expressed in the form of intense emotions. Strong emotions that are ignored or rejected by others, usually increase. Strong feelings recognized and accepted by others usually leads to decrease. Therefore, resistance is best met by curious exploration (Sommers-Flanagan et al., 2011). The social worker and the family will often experience it as an invitation to get to know each other in a respectful way instead of defining each other with labels, which often is a result of projection. Dwelling on the intense emotions and the content of resistance often mutes the intensity of the resistance if the counsellor holds an attitude of respect for the client's autonomy. An important responsibility for the supervisor is to hold focus on the process where the social worker establishes and maintains cooperation and look out for situations that can jeopardize the necessary collaboration for reaching the goal for the family.

To confirm intense feelings does not mean to encourage or accept physical acting-out, but to tolerate to some extent verbal outburst, but not accept threats. Supervisors can help professionals to use a meta-perspective on verbal outburst to handle them. As an example, a supervisee can be invited to consider how to approach their clients when they are more relaxed, and then to be more able to help them manage their loss of control. It can be discussed how this can be employed to help generalize to other situations in the future in other relationships.

Sometimes family members express strong emotions. One of the supervisor's tasks is to contain the feelings of the family members (or the social workers as well) by sorting them out together. One can do this by (1) hearing out the persons' feelings, (2) showing acceptance of them by commenting on them and (3) then one might interpret them. Professionals can learn a lot of whom they are by their own reactions to and understanding of the feelings of the family, like in an introspective way.

Intrinsic Instead of Extrinsic Motivation

It is an important step for families to move from extrinsic to intrinsic motivation to make changes—not because they must (social control), but because they want to change their life. Often social workers have an important influence on families to make that change of motivation, and it usually reduces the resistance against the CPS and the families tend to be more positive to receiving help. Extrinsic motivation easily maintains a position for the family feeling being of second class as they feel pressure to change in the direction of goals set by CPS. To change from extrinsic to intrinsic motivation for change assumes that the families can find meaning in the change, a form of "what's in it for me?".

Supervisors can support the social workers to find concern alliances with the family and emphasize this when forming goals for the change, e.g. by answering the questions: "What causes most stress for the family right now", "What is the family's idea of good life?", "Have the family tried to change some of their challenges, and succeeded or failed?", "What could be a goal for change that is not too difficult, but they will notice the difference?", "What kind of changes would probably lead to a significant difference", etc.

Intrinsic motivation remains an important construct, reflecting the natural human propensity to learn and assimilate. However, extrinsic motivation is argued to vary considerably in its relative autonomy and thus can either reflect external control or true self-regulation (Deci & Ryan, 2008a, 2008b, 2012; Ryan & Deci, 2017). Extrinsic motivation is a product of feeling one ought to or should, or external pressure or general expectations in the social network/society. It might help families to develop intrinsic motivation and reduce the resistance with support of the methods externalizing the problem and/or Motivational Interviewing (presented in this chapter). As the family change from extrinsic to intrinsic motivation, the resistance against the CPS usually reduces.

Motivational Interviewing (MI)

The mechanisms and effects of MI are similar to externalizing. Supervisor could suggest for the counsellor the use of motivational interviewing (MI) to help the client to clarify what is in it for them. The goal of MI is to engage client to change, clarify their strengths and possibilities, their aspirations that motivates them, as well as promote autonomy of decision making. The usefulness of MI is that it can lead to enhanced motivation to change and diminished resistance (Moyers & Rollnick, 2002). An emergent theory of MI is proposed that emphasizes two specific active components: A relational component focused on empathy and the interpersonal spirit of MI, and a technical component involving the differential evocation and reinforcement of client change talk (Miller & Rose, 2009).

MI can be useful for persons that suffer from different types of mental problems (Apodaca & Longbaugh, 2009; Armstrong et al., 2011; Lundahl, & Burke, 2009; McMurran, 2009; Miller & Rollnick, 2013; Rollnick et al., 2010). MI is not suitable for some of the most severe disorders, like psychosis/schizophrenia (Barrowclough et al., 2010). MI is a technique that is at its best when combined with evidence-based counselling methods or psychotherapies (Lundahl et al., 2010).

Suggestions for the Social Worker–Supervisor Relationship

Sometimes MI is useful for families to reflect on their contribution to the change. Supervisors could raise the awareness of the social workers how they by using questions from MI can facilitate families' motivation to change from defensive behaviour and extrinsic motivation to optimistic and often energetic behaviour and intrinsic motivation where the families take charge of the change processes.

Externalizing the Referral and the Standard Set by the CPS

It can be useful for the families if the social workers help the family to externalize the content of the referral and the problems. Instead of feeling hurt or angry because of the allegations in the referral, the social worker can help the family developing appropriate mastery strategies. Information in referrals is often diffuse, so the social worker can help the family in finding out the expectations of the professionals at CPS has for family functioning. The social worker can help the family to pick out strategies to work to meet the expectations of the CPS. The goal is to help the family to be offensive instead of defensive. Since the early 1990s, when being introduced to the work of narrative therapy by Michael White (1988, 1989), I have seen the usefulness of externalizing problems in conversations with counsellors and client. The notion is to talk about the problem as if it is distinct and separate from the person. Although it is aid that this treatment was first elaborated in work with children with encopresis, it has since been generalized for use with a wide range of problems and has been applied successfully in work with individual adults, couples and families. A relation of power imbalance and executing social control might be a bit balanced if the counsellor externalizes the demands from CPS. The family can use it as a target for anger, fear and hopelessness, as well as mobilizing energy and create strategies to solve problems. The social worker and the family can work together in the development of strategies and encourage each other to fight the problems. The concept of externalizing makes it possible for the social workers to collaborate with the families. The supervisor can be helpful for the social worker and the family in emphasizing the importance of being in an offensive position.

Externalizing techniques is within the narrative perspective (Roth & Epston, 1996a, 1996b). Examples of questions to be asked are: "If it was possible to do so, how would you like to limit the situation of being referred to this service instead of asking for it?", "Has this referral only influenced negatively on your self-esteem, or is there some positive aspects as well?", "Despite the situation and how you feel about it, how did you manage to defy these negative perceptions of the situation you have ended up with, and came for this conversation?", "What might this tell you about your abilities to fight against obstacles?", "In what other ways have you stood up for yourself and not let though situations overwhelm you?", "How long will you let the bad situation influence your life, and how ready are you to take further step against this situation that has such a grip on you?", "When will you end this unreasonable position that has muddled your life for a rather long time?", etc. Hopefully, questions like these invite the person to reflect and mobilize to take charge over their situation and life. Externalizing is sometimes motivating, but there is a balance between inviting the family to work together with the counsellor towards a goal and disguise the imbalance of power and social control. It blurs the boundaries that separate the two positions in an unethical way because they cannot ease. Probably will an attitude of warmth and a wish for helping, invite to collaboration despite the imbalance of power.

Working/Therapeutic Alliance

The therapeutic or working alliance between supervisor and supervised is important for establishing a trustful environment characterized by a safe atmosphere and openness, which makes it possible to stand by ones' uncertainty and doubts one might feel about the abilities they have to help people, frustrations, feeling pity for the client, etc. Even more important is the working alliance between social worker and client, because of non-equal power of the relation, the risk for persistent extrinsic motivation and enduring resistance.

Freud was the first one to conceptualize the notion of alliance. He postulated that the effective transference, and an analytic pact were necessary for the patient to hear the analyst's interpretations (Freud, 1912, 1937, here from Byerly, 1993; Shaughnessy, 1995). The term therapeutic alliance was introduced by Zetzel (1956), and the term working alliance was introduced by Greenson (1965, 1967).

Professionals and families usually have different opinions on the quality of alliance and what was the "turning points" for change (Kazdin 2007; Scholes et al. 2007), as well as scoring the quality of working alliance differently (Friedlander et al., 2006; Heinonen et al., 2014; McLeod & Weisz, 2005; Nissen-Lie et al., 2015). The advice is to include evaluations from the clients and willingness to negotiate changes of contents of the sessions (Flückiger et al., 2011; Lambert & Shimokawa, 2011). The concept of working alliance is not to be interpreted as static, as it changes during the period of counselling (Creed & Kendall, 2005; McLeod, 2009). Supervisors wisely encourage the social workers to talk on regular basis with the families about the working alliance to be able to judge the quality of it and adjust the content or form of the counselling.

Suggestions for the Social Worker–Supervisor Relationship

The bulky amount of research on the effects of working alliance in counselling and psychotherapy highlights the importance of working alliance between counsellor and clients, and as a consequence this ought to be one of the main themes in supervision, i.e. focus on the social workers working alliances with the families (Arnow et al., 2013; Baldwin & Imel, 2013; Del Re et al., 2012; Flückiger et al. 2012; Laska et al., 2014; Sly et al., 2014; Wampold, 2015; Zaitsoff et al., 2015). Working alliance is held to be of greater importance than specific techniques used or the frequency of sessions or duration of treatment (Norcross 2010; Wampold, 2015; Wampold & Imel, 2015a, 2015b). It seems as if the characteristics of the social worker are of greater importance for the effect of the professional conversations, than characteristics of the client (Marcus et al., 2011; Zuroff et al., 2010). In sum: Factors, such as the working alliance, empathy, expectations, psychoeducation about the problems, and other so-called common factors, are robustly related to outcome of interventions. Moreover, and importantly, those therapists who can form an alliance with a range of patients have a sophisticated set of facilitative interpersonal skills, worry about their effectiveness and make deliberate efforts to improve are the counsellors who achieve better outcomes (Wampold & Imel, 2015a, b).

Supervisors need to form working alliances with those supervised, as well as the professionals should form strong working alliance to their clients. As a supervisor, one could inspire and guide the social workers to establish a strong working alliance with their families based on the research on what tends to form these strong connections (i.e. Oddli & Rønnestad, 2012; Hawamdeh & Fakhry, 2014; Håvås et al., 2015; Malin & Pos, 2015; Watson et al., 2014): (1) an outspoken interest to know the client, (2) expressions of warmth and empathy, (3) an acceptance for what the person is and the thoughts, feelings and behaviour, (4) being active instead of passive/receptive, (5) support of the client's self-agency (facilitate processes for making decisions, believing in oneself and taking actions), (6) being optimistic on the behalf of the client, (7) matching of the clients' nonverbal expressions, (8) responding sensitive to the talks of the client and (9) helping the client with practical tasks: checking out, getting information, making decisions, etc., to show power of action and that one wants to be helpful.

Supervisors can influence the counsellor's ability and awareness of the importance of establishing solid working alliance with the families by having this as a topic in most of the supervisions. The background of the counsellor influences their ability to establish working alliances (Heinonen et al., 2014; Hersoug et al., 2009; Nissen-Lie et al., 2013).

The attachment of the counsellor influences their ability to form working alliances (Dinger et al., 2009; Wyatt-Brooks, 2013). The effect size between the attachment of the counsellor and how easy they form working alliances to clients is moderate (Ryan et al., 2012). Social workers can learn some of the skills that nurtures working alliances, even though professionals vary in competence for establishing working alliances. The effect size between the attachment of the counsellor and how social workers that manage to form solid working alliances to a variety of clients is explained by their capacity of mentalization, social competence and attachment quality (Anderson et al., 2010).

Even though working alliance, empathy and warmth are some of the corner stones for the relationship between counsellors and clients, the literature warns against empathy being too strong (Fog & Hem, 2009; Ulvik & Rønnestad, 2013). Excessive identification with the client leads the counsellor easily slips on the target of the conversations and alternative options (Fog & Hem, 2009; Ulvik & Rønnestad, 2013). Supervisors have an important role of discovering when the counsellor struggles with balancing empathy and warmth with necessary distance. The awareness of this dilemma seems to help several counsellors to adjust their thinking of the client and behaviour.

Attachment Theory and Supervision: Building Trust

Working alliances is influenced by the person sense of knowing what things mean and what is true: epistemic trust or epistemic distrust.[3] Epistemic dis-/trust is connected to attachment and mentalization (Bernier et al., 2014; Daley, 2013; Fonagy & Allison, 2014). One might say that epistemic trust is trust in communication and to pull bills of exchange on other people's experiences and reflections. As exploring is a central part of attachment, persons with secure attachment score in general the working alliance to the professional as better than persons with insecure attachments (Liotti, 2004; Smith et al., 2010). The consequence is that persons with insecure attachments are in higher risk for drop-out from counselling compared to persons with secure attachments (McLeod, 2011; Shorey & Snyder, 2006).

Supervisors as Secure Base and Safe Haven

According to the concept of Circle of Security (CoS), professionals can be the secure base and the safe haven for parents or children. This is illustrated by two hands at one of the ends of the circle (Powell et al., 2013). The basic assumption of the model is that the counsellor acts like

---

[3] In dictionaries, episteme is defined as intellectually certain knowledge/the body of ideas that determine the knowledge that is intellectually certain at any particular time. The word epistemic is originating from the Greek *epistēmē* understanding, knowledge, from feminine of *epistēmōn* understanding, knowing, from *epistanai* to understand, know, from *epi-+ histanai* to set, place.

"hands" for the parents in order to inspire them to be the hands for their children.

According to CoS, one uses the metaphor of a seesaw. When a person is up on the top of the circle, they are feeling safe and are in modus for exploring, learning and creativity. It is often useful if parents in interactions with their children show (1) that they watch over them, (2) delight in them, (3) helping them and (4) enjoy with them. It is useful for parents if social workers show the same principles of interactions.

Several times each and every day persons feel like being down on the circle because they are unsure of situation and/or situation, e.g. have negative feelings, failed, are exhausted, etc. According to the seesaw, when children are down on the circle, they are in the need of parents that (1) protect them, (2) comfort them, (3) have delight in them and (4) organize their feelings. When parents feel like being down on the circle, it can be relational strengthening if the social workers show this form of care for them.

Suggestions for the Social Worker–Supervisor Relationship

In the same way as social workers are inspiring hands for children, it often is fruitful if supervisors show care for social workers in the same manner. Professionals can be on the top as well as at the bottom of the circle: They can feel competent and master situations, as well as feeling shame as they do not master the situations as they want to or what is expected from them, and they feel discouraged and abandoned. For the latter, they need to be comforted and understood by the supervisor as well as encouraged. For the former, they need an engaged supervisor that join them and express delight in them, joy and pride on behalf of their stories. As for working alliances and the need for confirming intense emotions, there is mutual relational processes between supervisors and supervised, as it is between professionals and their families according to needs whether one is on top of or bottom of the circle.

Concluding Remarks

Especially inexperienced social workers tend to overrate the effect of methods/programmes, exaggerate the clients' resources and minimalize the clients' difficulties, as well as too much confidence in the effect of methods (Rønnestad & Skovholt, 2003). Counsellors can be vulnerable to becoming overwhelmed with responsibility and feelings of inadequacy, isolation and despair (Råbu et al., 2016). For many professionals, the first (often five) years in the working life can be a challenge. Supervisors could help professionals making realistic assessments of the families and cooperate with them in the planning of how to include family members and set reachable goals and suitable interventions.

Supervision is complex social processes, at least on two levels: Managing/containing the complex feelings that social workers face due to their work tasks and helping social workers to develop and utilize theory, to impart results from empirical research and initiate processes of reflection. This includes the following elements: (1) Discussions with the social workers, (2) use of psychoeducational elements (primarily based on empirical studies, but sometimes theories), (3) rehearsal on microcompetencies (e.g. in what way they could ask questions, how to invite to collaboration, how to establish "alliances built on common concern", etc.) and (4) being a role model for the social workers of how they can cooperate with families.

Transparency and involvement are the key issues to create intrinsic motivation in family members which often reduces the resistance. The combination of helping families and at the same time exercise social control might foster suspicion which leads to resistance. The responsibility rests on the professionals to create a fruitful cooperation with the families. They have to take most of the initiatives to reduce families' resistance, because resistance often leads to withdrawal or outbursts and not cooperation.

Supervising workers in the CPS are a relational process with clear parallels to the professionals contact with families: Establishing working alliances that endures hard times, supporting when families feel like being on the top of the circle and comforting when they are at the bottom of the circle, as well as finding strength in intrinsic motivation for the job that needs to be done. Humans have in common the need to be in relation to others, they need to feel confident because they feel respected and understood by people that master to contain their feelings, encourages them to reach their goals, developing competence and enhancing their self-esteem. It is pretty much all about achieving and protecting one's dignity.

References

Andersen, T. (1996). Language is not innocent. In F. W. Kaslow (Ed.), *Wiley series in couples and family dynamics and treatment. Handbook of relational diagnosis and dysfunctional family patterns* (pp. 119–125). Wiley.

Anderson, T., Lunnen, K. M., & Ogles, B. M. (2010). Putting models and techniques in context. In B. L. Duncan, S. D. Miller, B. E. Wampold, & M. A. Hubble (Eds.), *The heart and soul of change: Delivering what works in therapy* (pp. 143–166). Washington DC: American Psychological Association.

Apodaca, T. R., & Longbaugh, R. (2009). Mechanisms of change in motivational interviewing: A review and preliminary evaluation of the evidence. *Addiction, 104*(5), 705–715. https://doi.org/10.1111/j.1360-0443.2009.02527.x.

Armstrong, M. J., Mottershead, T. A., Ronksley, P. E., Sigal, R. J., Campbell, T. S., & Hemmelgarn, B. R. (2011). Motivational interviewing to improve weight loss in overweight and/or obese patients: A systematic review and meta-analysis of randomized controlled trials. *Obesity Reviews, 12*(9), 709–723. https://doi.org/10.1111/j.1467-789x.2011.00892.x.

Arnow, B. A., Constantino, M. J., Klein, D. N., Markowitz, J. C., Rothbaum, J. C., Thase, M. E., et al. (2013). The relationship between the therapeutic alliance and treatment outcome in two distinct psychotherapies for chronic depression. *Journal of Consulting and Clinical Psychology, 81*(4), 627–638. https://doi.org/10.1037/a0031530.

Baldwin, S. A., & Imel, Z. E. (2013). Therapist effects: Finding and methods. In M. J. Lambert (Ed.), *Bergin and Garfield's handbook of psychotherapy and behavior change* (6th ed., pp. 258–297). Wiley.

Barrowclough, C., Haddock, G., Wykes, T., Beardmore, R., Conrod, P., Craig, T., et al. (2010). Integrated motivational interviewing and cognitive behavioural therapy for people with psychosis and comorbid substance misuse: Randomised controlled trial. *British Medical Journal, 341,*. https://doi.org/10.1136/bmj.c6325.

Bernier, A., Matte-Gagné, C., Bélanger, M.-E., & Whipple, N. (2014). Taking stock of two decades of attachment transmission gap: Broadening the assessment of maternal behavior. *Child Development, 85,* 1852–1865.

Byerly, L. J. (1993). The therapeutic alliance. In H. Etezady (Ed.), *Treatment of neurosis in the young: A psychoanalytic perspective* (pp. 19–50). Jason Aronson.

Creed, T. A., & Kendall, P. C. (2005). Therapist alliance-building behavior within a cognitive-behavioral treatment for anxiety in youth. *Journal of Consulting and Clinical Psychology, 73*(3), 498–505. https://doi.org/10.1037/0022-006X.73.3.498.

Daley, E. (2013). *Reflective functioning and differentiation-relatedness during pregnancy and infant attachment outcomes at one year* (Ph.D. thesis at The City University of New York).

Deci, E. L., & Ryan, R. M. (2008a). Facilitating optimal motivation and psychological well-being across life's domains. *Canadian Psychology/Psychologie Canadienne, 49*(3), 14–23. https://doi.org/10.1037/0708-5591.49.1.14.

Deci, E. L., & Ryan, R. M. (2008b). Self-determination theory: A macrotheory of human motivation, development, and health. *Canadian Psychology/Psychologie Canadienne, 49*(3), 182–185. https://doi.org/10.1037/a0012801.

Deci, E. L., & Ryan, R. M. (2012). Motivation, personality, and development within embedded social contexts: An overview of self-determination theory. In R. M. Ryan (Ed.), *Oxford handbook of human motivation* (pp. 85–107). Oxford University Press.

Del Re, A. C., Flückiger, C., Horvath, A. O., Symonds, D. & Wampold, B. E. (2012). Therapist effects in the therapeutic alliance-outcome relationship: A restrictedmaximum likelihood meta-analysis. *Clinical Psychology Review, 32*(7), 642–649. http://doi.org/10.1111/j.1468-2850.2009.01145.x.

DeRubeis, R. J., Gelfand, L. A., German, R. E., Fournier, J. C., & Forand, N. C. (2014). Understanding processes of change: How some patients reveal more than others—And some groups of therapists less—About what matters in psychotherapy. *Psychotherapy Research, 24*(3), 419–428.

Dinger, U., Strack, M., Sachsse, T., & Schauenberg, H. (2009). Therapists' attachment, patients' interpersonal problems and alliance development over

time in inpatient psychotherapy. *Psychotherapy: Theory, Research, Practice, Training*, *46*(3), 277–290. https://doi.org/10.1037/a0016913.
Flückiger, C., Del Re, A. C., Wampold, B. E., Symonds, D., & Horvath, A. O (2012). How central is the alliance in psychotherapy? A multilevel longitudinal meta-analysis. *Journal of Counseling Psychology*, *59*(1), 10–17.
Flückiger, C., Meyer, A., Wampold, B. E., Gassmann, D., Messerli-ürgy, N., & Munsch, S. (2011). Predicting premature termination within a randomized controlled trial for binge-eating patients. *Behavior Therapy*, *42*(4), 716–725.
Fog, J., & Hem, L. (2009). *Psykoterapi og erkendelse. Personligty anliggende og profesonel virksomhed* [*Psychotherapy and recognition. Privacy and business*]. Akademisk Forlag.
Fonagy, P., & Allison, E. (2014). The role of mentalizing and epistemic trust in the therapeutic relationship. *Psychotherapy*, *51*(3), 372–380. https://doi.org/10.1037/a0036505.
Freud, S. (1912). *The dynamics of the transference*. Hogarth Press.
Freud, S. (1937). *Analysis terminable and interminable*. Hogarth Press.
Friedlander, M. L., Escudero, V., & Heatherington, L. (2006). *Therapeutic alliances in couple and family therapy: An empirically informed guide to practice*. American Psychological Association. https://doi.org/10.1037/114 10-000.
Greenson, R. R. (1965). The working alliance and the transference neurosis. *Psychoanalytic Quarterly*, *34*, 155–181.
Greenson, R. R. (1967). *The technique and practice of psychoanalysis* (Vol. 1). International Universities Press.
Hawamdeh, S., & Fakhry, R. (2014). Therapeutic relationships from the psychiatric nurses' perspectives: An interpretative phenomenological study. *Perspectives in Psychiatric Care*, *50*(3), 178–185. https://doi.org/10.1111/ppc.12039.
Heinonen, E., Lindfors, O., Härkänen, T., Virtala, E., Jääskeläinen, T., & Knekt, P. (2014). Therapists' professional and personal characteristics as predictors of working alliance in short-term and long-term psychotherapies. *Clinical Psychology & Psychotherapy*, *21*(6), 475–494. https://doi.org/10.1002/cpp.1852.
Hersoug, A. G., Høglend, P., Havik, O., von der Lippe, A., & Monsen, J. (2009). Therapist characteristics influencing the quality of alliance in long-term psychotherapy. *Clinical Psychology & Psychotherapy*, *16*(2), 100–110. https://doi.org/10.1002/cpp.605.

Håvås, E., Svartberg, M., & Ulvenes, P. (2015). Attuning to the unspoken: The relationship between therapist nonverbal attunement and attachment security in adult psychotherapy. *Psychoanalytiuc Psychology, 32*(2), 235–254.

Kazdin, A. E. (2007). Mediators and mechanisms of change in psychotherapy research. *Annual Review of Clinical Psychology, 3*, 1–27. https://doi.org/10.1146/annurev.clinpsy.3.02806.091432.

Kazdin, A. E., Whitley, M., & Marciano, P. L. (2006). Child–therapist and parent–therapist alliance and therapeutic change in the treatment of children referred for oppositional, aggressive, and antisocial behavior. *Journal of Child Psychology and Psychiatry, 47*(5), 436–445. https://doi.org/10.1111/j.1469-7610.2005.01475.x.

Lambert, M. J., & Shimokawa, K. (2011). Collecting client feedback. *Psychotherapy, 48*(1), 72–79. https://doi.org/10.1037/a0022238.

Lambert, M. J., & Simon, W. (2008). The therapeutic relationship: Central and essential psychotherapy outcome. In S. F. Hick & T. Bien (Eds.), *Mindfulness and the therapeutic relationship* (pp. 19–33). The Guilford Press.

Laska, K. M., Gurman, A. S., & Wampold, B. E. (2014). Expanding the lens of evidence-based practice in psychotherapy: A common factors perspective. *Psychotherapy, 51*(4), 467–481.

Lazarus, G., Atzil-Slonim, D., Bar-Kalifa, E., Hasson-Ohayon, I., & Rafaeli, E. (2019). Clients' emotional instability and therapists' inferential flexibility predict therapists' session-by-session empathic accuracy. *Journal of Counseling Psychology, 66*(1), 56–69. https://doi.org/10.1037/cou0000310.

Liotti, G. (2004). Trauma, dissociation, and disorganized attachment: Three strands of a single braid. *Psychotherapy: Theory, Research, Practice, Training, 41*(4), 472–486. https://doi.org/10.1037/0033-3204.41.4.472.

Lundahl, B., & Burke, B. L. (2009). The effectiveness and applicability of motivational interviewing: A practice-friendly review of four meta-analyses. *Journal of Clinical Psychology, 65*(11), 1232–1245. https://doi.org/10.1002/jclp.20638.

Lundahl, B. W., Kunz, C., Brownell, C., Tollefson, D., & Burke, B. L. (2010). A meta-analysis of motivational interviewing: Twenty-five years of empirical studies. *Research on Social Work Practice, 20*(2), 137–160. https://doi.org/10.1177/1049731509347850.

Manthorpe, J., Moriarty, J., Hussein, S., Stevens, M., & Sharpe, E. (2013). Content and purpose of supervision in social work practice in England: Views of newly qualified social workers, managers and directors. *British Journal of Social Work, 45*(1), 52–68. https://doi.org/10.1093/bjsw/bct102.

Malin, A. J., & Pos, A. E. (2015). The impact of early empathy on alliance building, emotional processing, and outcome during experiential treatment of depression. *Psychotherapy Research, 25*(4), 445–459. https://doi.org/10.1080/10503307.2014.901572.

Marcus, M., Westra, H., Angus, L., & Kertes, A. (2011). Client experiences of motivational interviewing for generalized anxiety disorder: A qualitative analysis. *Psychotherapy Research, 21*(4), 447–461. https://doi.org/10.1080/10503307.2011.578265.

Martinsen, E., & Lichtwarck, W. (2013). *Det nye barnevernet* [The new child protection service]. Universitetsforlaget.

McLeod, B. D. (2009). Understanding why therapy allegiance is linked to clinical outcomes. *Clinical Psychology Science and Practice, 16*(1), 69–72. https://doi.org/10.1111/j.1468-2850.2009.01145.x.

McLeod, B. D. (2011). Relation of the alliance with outcomes in youth psychotherapy: A meta-analysis. *Clinical Psychology Review, 31*(4), 603–616. https://doi.org/10.1016/j.cpr.2011.02.001.

McLeod, B. D., & Weisz, J. R. (2005). The therapy process observational coding system-alliance scale: Measure characteristics and prediction of outcome in usual clinical practice. *Journal of Consulting and Clinical Psychology, 73*(2), 323–333. https://doi.org/10.1037/0022-006X.73.2.323.

McMurran, M. (2009). Motivational interviewing with offenders: A systematic review. *Legal and Criminological Psychology, 14*(1), 83–100. https://doi.org/10.1348/135532508x278326.

Miller, W. R., & Rollnick, S. (2013). *Motivational interviewing: Helping people change*. The Guilford Press.

Miller, W. R., & Rose, G. S. (2009). Toward a theory of motivational interviewing. *American Psychologist, 64*(6), 527–537. https://doi.org/10.1037/a0016830.

Moyers, T. B., & Rollnick, S. (2002). A motivational interviewing perspective on resistance in psychotherapy. *Psychotherapy in Practice, 58*(2), 185–193. https://doi.org/10.1002/jclp.1142.

Murphy, R., Cooper, Z., Hollon, S. D., & Fairburn, C. G. (2009). How do psychological treatments work? Investigating mediators of change? *Behaviour Research and Therapy, 47*(1), 1–5. https://doi.org/10.1016/j.brat.2008.10.001.

Nissen-Lie, H. A., Havik, O. E., Høglend, P. A., Rønnestad, M. H., & Monsen, J. T. (2015). Patient and therapist perspectives on alliance development: Therapists' practice experiences as predictors. *Clinical Psychology & Psychotherapy, 22*(4), 317–327. https://doi.org/10.1002/cpp.1891.

Nissen-Lie, H. A., Monsen, J. T., Ulleberg, P., & Rønnestad, M. H. (2013). Psychotherapists' self-reports of their interpersonal functioning and difficulties in practice as predictors of patient outcome. *Psychotherapy Research, 23*(1), 86–104. https://doi.org/10.1080/10503307.2012.735775.

Norcross, J. C., & Wampold, B. E. (2010). What works for whom: Tailoring psychotherapy to the person. *Journal of Clinical psychology, 67*(2), 127–132. https://doi.org/10.1002/jclp.20764.

Oddli, H., & Rønnestad, M. H. (2012). How experienced therapists introduce the technical aspects in the initial alliance formation: Powerful decision makers supporting clients' agency. *Psychotherapy Research, 22*(2), 176–193. https://doi.org/10.1080/10503307.2011.633280.

Powell, B., Cooper, G., Hoffman, K., & Marvin, R. (2013). *The Circle of Security Intervention: Enhancing attachment in early parent-child relationships*. The Guilford Press.

Rollnick, S., Butler, C. C., Kinnersley, P., Gregory, J., & Mash, B. (2010). Competent novice: Motivational interviewing. *British Medical Journal, 340*(5), 1242–1245.

Roth, S. & Epston, D. (1996a). Developing externalizing conversations: An exercise. *Journal of Systemic Therapies, 15*(1), 5–12.

Roth, S., & Epston, D. (1996b). Consulting the problem about the problematic relationship: An exercise for experiencing a relationship with an externalized problem. In M. Hoyt (Ed.), *Constructive therapies* (Vol. 2, pp. 148–162). The Guilford Press.

Ryan, A., Safran, J. D., Doran, J. M., & Derner, J. C. M. (2012). Therapist mindfulness, alliance, and treatment outcome. *Psychotherapy Research, 22*(3), 289–297. https://doi.org/10.1080/10503307.2011.650653.

Ryan, R. M., & Deci, E. L. (2017). *Self-determination theory: Basic psychological needs in motivation, development, and wellness*. The Guilford Press.

Rynn, M., Khalid-Khan, S., Garcia-Espana, J. F., Etemad, B., & Rickels, K. (2006). Early response and 8-week treatment outcome in GAD. *Depression and Anxiety, 23*(8), 461–465. https://doi.org/10.1002/da.20214.

Rønnestad, M. H., & Skovholt, T. M. (2003). The journey of the counselor and therapist: Research findings and perspectives on professional development. *Journal of Career Development, 30*(1), 5–44.

Råbu, M., Moltu, C., Binder, P.-E., & McLeod, J. (2016). How does practicing psychotherapy affect the personal life of the therapist? A qualitative inquiry of senior therapists' experiences. *Psychotherapy Research, 26*(6), 737–749.

Shaughnessy, P. (1995). Empathy and the working alliance: The mistranslation of Freud's Einfuhlung. *Psychoanalytic Psychology, 12,* 221–231. https://doi.org/10.1111/j.1752-0606.2004.tb01229.x.

Shorey, H. S., & Snyder, C. R. (2006). The role of adult attachment styles in psychopathology and psychotherapy outcomes. *Review of General psychology, 10*(1), 1–20. https://doi.org/10.1037/1089-2680.10.1.1.

Sly, R., Morgan, J. F., Mountford, V. A., Sawer, F., Evans, C., & Lacey, J. H. (2014). Rules of engagement: Qualitative experiences of therapeutic alliance when receiving in-patient treatment for Anorexia Nervosa. *Eating Disorders, 22*(3), 233–243. https://doi.org/10.1080/10640266.2013.867742.

Smith, A. E. M., Msetfi, R. M., & Golding, L. (2010). Client self rated adult attachment patterns and the therapeutic alliance: A systematic review. *Clinical Psychology Review, 30*(3), 326–337.

Sommers-Flanagan, J., Richardson, B. G., & Sommers-Flanagan, R. (2011). A multi-theoretical, evidence-based approach for understanding and managing adolescent resistance to psychotherapy. *Journal of Contemporary Psychotherapy, 41*(2), 69–80. https://doi.org/10.1007/s10879-010-9164-y.

Ulvik, O. S., & Rønnestad, M. H. (2013). Cultural discourses of helping: Perspectives on what people bring with them when they start training in therapy and counseling. In M. H. Rønnestad & T. M. Skovholt (Eds.), *The developing practitioner: Growth and stagnation of therapists and counselors* (pp. 37–52). Routledge.

Wampold, B. E. (2015). How important are the common factors in psychotherapy? An update. *World Psychiatry, 14*(3), 270–277. https://doi.org/10.1002/wps.20238.

Wampold, B., & Imel, Z. E. (2015a). *The great psychotherapy debate. The evidence for what makes psychotherapy work.* Routledge.

Wampold, B., & Imel, Z. (2015b). *What do we know about psychotherapy?—And what is there left to debate?* http://www.societyforpsychotherapy.org/what-do-we-know-about-psychotherapy-and-what-is-there-left-to-debate.

Watson, J. C., Steckley, P. L., & McMullen, E. J. (2014). The role of empathy in promoting change. *Psychotherapy Research, 24*(3), 286–298. https://doi.org/10.1080/10503307.2013.802823.

White, M. (1988). The externalizing of the problem and the re-authoring of lives and relationships. In M. White (Ed.), *Selected papers* (pp. 5–28). Dulwich Centre Publications.

White, M. (1989). Pseudo-encopresis: From avalanche to victory, from vicious to virtuous cycles. In M. White (Ed.), *Selected papers* (pp. 115–124). Dulwich Centre Publications.

Wyatt-Brooks, K. (2013). *The association between therapists' attachment security and mentalizing capacity* (Ph.D. at University College London).

Zaitsoff, S., Pullmer, R., Cyr, M., & Aime, H. (2015). The role of the therapeutic alliance in eating disorder treatment outcomes: A systematic review. *Eating Disorders, 23*(2), 99–114. https://doi.org/10.1080/10640266.2014.964623.

Zetzel, E. R. (1956). Current concepts of transference. *International Journal of Psycho-Analysis, 37*, 369–376.

Zuroff, D. C., Kelly, A. C., Leybman, M. J., Blatt. S. J., & Wampold, B. E. (2010). Between-therapist and within-therapist mdifferences in the quality of the therapeutic relationship: Effects on maladjustment and self-critical perfectionism. *Journal of Clinical Psychology, 66*(7), 681–697.

6

The Artistry of Stuck-Ness

Billy Hardy

Introduction

In this chapter, I write about stuck-ness from a relational orientation and in the context of being stuck in supervisory relationships. The unintended consequence of the invitation to stuck-ness is that I become frozen in the moment as the multiple possibilities whiz through my head. This, of course, can fall many ways, like a deck of opened cards when considering the position I adopt to keep the conversation going.

A relational approach, as I argue, focuses on co-creation, interactional processes, supervisory alliances and how we create, learn, develop, and find a way to continue our conversations and practices. Equally, being stuck draws me to question how many moments of my practice I reveal, since it seems that being stuck is an everyday process of providing supervision, regardless of the varying contexts (with teams, individuals and public, private and not-for-profit organizations). Various questions come

B. Hardy (✉)
Centre for Systemic Studies, Wales, UK

to mind, and the song by Stealers wheel Stuck in the middle with you (1974). The song dates back to the 1970s. Some of a particular age will recognize it, and when you hear it in the future, you might think of this chapter.

As I think about addressing the issue of being stuck in a supervisory context, I wonder how I should position myself. Shall I write about getting stuck in supervision as a therapist or as a supervisor? Shall I take up another position such as being stuck as a training supervisor for a clinical training course in the postgraduate training of family therapists? Shall I take the position of a supervisor outside of a training context, maybe with a team, an agency or in my private practice?

The other important consideration is that supervisees may, at times, be stuck with you as a supervisor and the challenges that arise from working with stuck supervisors. As you can see, there are several options with which to work or play. Stuck-ness in supervision is multi-layered and multi-textured. It is likely a mixture of different positions in different contexts with different folks. I suggest this as my supervisory practices cut across different contexts, skill levels, orientations, and of course many opportunities for getting stuck. I am, for the most part, stuck with being stuck, and this has increased over time as I gather more and more experiences, particularly in supervisory relationships.

On a personal note, one of these stuck processes is the fact that, as I type this, I can barely use my right hand (*I am right-handed*) as I am currently in the middle of osteopathic treatment to unlock my stuck shoulder and my forefinger and thumb are frozen. Maybe, a bit more on that later.

I am also interested in what lies outside of the confines of supervisory relationships and what I can bring into the domain of supervisory practice to enrich and expand repertoires for myself and that of others, who may often present with a stuck case, problem, context or dilemma. The variety of contexts will, in themselves, be challenges, as will a micro-moment in therapy, a difficult theoretical position to get used to, a legal challenge, a learning challenge, a team challenge, and the list continues. I attempt to bring a set of relational markers; markers that are less concerned with the supervisory theory and more focused on theories of learning that have been personally useful and sometimes creative. When

I speak of creativity, I draw upon Keeney's (2014) definition. He says creativity is "a process metaphor for a radical constructivist view that emphasizes invention, construction, improvisation and creation" (p. 3).

The song was chosen for the specific reason that it implies creativity in different spheres. First, what do I do in the middle with whom? Second, clowns are positioned on the left of me and this is a good thing because, as you know, being a clown takes a lot of training, creativity and improvisation. I was lucky to experience this at a study centre I attended. I happened to bump into a group who were training to be clowns and, much like other forms of practice, the degree of sophistication and learning was much like being a supervisor working with a live team. Finally, jokers on the right of me and, are also creative and work hard, rehearse, build materials and, of course, improvise. The song captures the team focus and artistry required of me, my colleagues and trainees.

Three other significant dimensions and characters thread through this chapter: jazz, dance (GAGA) improvisation and the art of avoiding the "blah blah, blah" (Friere, 2001). The three positions will be connected with the art of teaching and learning as presented by Barry Harris (YouTube, 2019). His inspirational class on working with the "and space" between notes (e.g., 1,2,3,4 "and") resonates with this chapter. Resonance also emerges from Ohad Naharin's (2016) dance-but-not-dance Gaga method. Naharin is a choreographer who also inspired my discussion on being stuck. Finally, blah blah blah is an acknowledgement of Paulo Friere's ideas. He said, "critical reflection on practice is a requirement of the relationship between theory and practice. Otherwise, theory becomes simply 'blah, blah, blah' and practice, pure activism" (Freire, 2001, p. 30).

I will attempt to uncover, explore, create and unfold the possibilities open to us when we are at an impasse, crossroad, cul-de-sac or going around the roundabout as we are faced with challenges that seem insurmountable in the moment. It is in moments like these that practitioners often think, "my supervisor will know what to do". Jones (2003), Laughlin (2000) and Telfener (2016) offer a myriad of possibilities for noticing, attending and creating contexts to unstick ourselves and colleagues who seek our views and ideas as supervisors. These may seem like familiar moments as you practice as a supervisor and your student wants to know what to do next. The answer may be on the tip of your tongue or you may have the luxury of a few moments to pause and reflect. You are skilled in the art of resistance or, as Gianfranco Cecchin would say, "do not understand too quickly".

The literature on clinical supervision continues to grow as a technical and rational process (Schon, 1987). It has a propensity for growing many new models to be codified, quantifying relationships in our professional lives, particularly in the so-called helping professions (i.e. the psych-oriented practices).

In many different countries, there are different rules, different legislation and governance for supervision and supervisors with expectations that supervisors will strictly follow and comply with these rules. For many, this is one of the distinguishing features of professional practice. In some countries, there may be a looser definition, unlegislated, more ethically oriented, more relationally bound perhaps, more embodied rather that espoused. Whichever the context of the practice or country of practice and the specific working arena, I would suggest we all know when we are stuck; we know when our supervisees are stuck. And, we have the responsibility to respond at the moment if we are practising live or sometimes we have the luxury of time in a retrospective mode. It is possibly one of the universals of the work we do, like driving a car. At some point, maybe depending upon where you live, you will end up in a traffic jam and be stuck.

Being Stuck. What Is It?

I aver that being stuck is, perhaps, less about being paralysed and more about what do we do next and how. Being stuck is a moment that invites us to ask how we might collaborate, negotiate and become creative so we might be able to shift to another possibility. This is akin to Vygotsky's (2007) zones of proximal development. By collaborating, we might be able to steer clear of constraints. How do we know what to do next whilst simultaneously respecting the therapist and client? What follows is a fragmentary moment in practice and the responses I make whilst holding a relational orientation.

Vignette 1

A trainee is working with a family, and it is a live supervisory context. It seems the trainee is running out of conversation. I notice this. There is a tension in the air. The members of the training team are on edge and the clients are looking puzzled. How do I respond and what do I need to consider? Who is the therapist in the moment? What level of experience does s/he have? What are my ethical considerations in this moment? The clients know we are offering the Milan/systemic process and the team is behind the screen. They also know that the team and the supervisor have a telephone link to the therapist. I have two options: (i) phone through and ask the therapist to come for a consultation, which is part of the practice culture or (ii) suggest that the therapist ask the family if they would like to hear from the team behind the screen. I take the latter option. The family agrees and the therapist is relieved. We swap rooms and the therapist joins the family who are now behind the screen.

We use a reflecting team process. In this moment of stuck-ness, as a clinical supervisor, I exercise my clinical responsibility in a relational frame. I speak with the clinical team as the family and therapist observe us. The process of conversation is now reversed, transparent and collaborative. Central here is holding the therapy in mind, holding the therapist in mind and holding the team in mind. I use the term mind in a Batesonian sense (1972)—"mind is social"—it is contextual and relational and requires a sensitivity to all within the conversational space we have created.

I offer words that acknowledge the tentative nature of the conversation thus far between the therapist and the family members. I sit with the moment of what to do next. There are contributions from the team, which come from an appreciative position.

We speak for no more than 5 minutes and we hope that what we have said might puncture the impasse being experienced by the novice therapist. The family and therapist return to the therapy room and continue their conversation. The therapist now has a renewed curiosity and confidence in his/her ability to start a dialogue with the family. We have offered the therapist some ideas for continuing the conversation and the family also picks up on the words offered by the reflecting team. The session ends with the offer of a new appointment and a comment about how they found the team's ideas useful.

This is one example of being stuck. As the supervisor, I was stuck. The therapist and the family were stuck. We were all stuck. However, in that moment, the training context provided the scaffolding to support this. Chen and Noodbond (1999) remind us of the complexity of the group or team process and offer a number of key ideas for what we call scaffolding. These are familiar, but often can be forgotten: both/and versus either/or. This idea has the potential to unfreeze seemingly intractable situations. In addition, engaging in an internal dialogue that is marked by humility and being specific and careful in offering feedback can aid connection with others. It is also useful to speak the unspeakable or leave the silence to speak. All of these and more may form part of the negotiated scaffolding of the team or group.

These will enrich the context. It is also not insignificant that the team has worked together for a long time. We have trust in my systemic relational "thermometer" and the team knows that I am constantly checking the relational temperature. Looking out for relational frames, possibilities for change and observing how meaning unfolds (Pearce, 2005). The trust, the focus on the possibility of change, and the close observation of the meaning-making process take place in the intimacy behind a screen where the focus is tense, demanding and challenges our emotional and relational abilities to stay with the dialogues in the therapy room. It may also be part of our ongoing teamwork with colleagues in a variety of working contexts, thereby forming part of the team process.

Through another lens, the actions of the supervisor may seem like a mistake, an error in process. However, these situations require learning in the moment. Another supervisor may choose a different intervention option; his/her position in these moments is multilayered and multitextured. Theories abound within the team, but offering a response is key to supporting the learning and the therapeutic process for the clients. These moments of feeling stuck offer trainees the chance to enter into a common process without fear of criticism or competition from the team. It helps avoid the "advisory" position (i.e. "this is what I would do") and, instead, engenders a search for a more appreciative positioning, particularly in the learning context.

From Gaga to Blah Blah. Ohad Naharin (2016), a choreographer of the GAGA method, described his practice as a context that is created so that errors can be made but held. The context created is the safety net for this to happen. The studio where his dancers meet and learn are provided with this safety net. Naharin is like the relationally attuned supervisor—highly skilled in the art of context creation. The scaffolding provides this sort of safety net as part of the learning process in therapy. The therapist, like Naharin's dancers, has the opportunity to experience their bodies and their responses in the presence of others who can support and develop how they can respond in these moments.

They can also appreciate that these processes will happen in and out of training, in their everyday practice with families. Naharin offers us the possibility of noticing that these processes are not only relational but physical. There is a self-reflexive loop between you, your own skin and your bones. The recognition that relationally oriented supervisors have the same structures as our supervisees can be liberating. Equally, our clients are connected to us. Recognizing this can also be seen, felt and heard in the work of Barry Harris (2012) who emphasizes the "ands", or the space between; an almost liminal space felt by many but can easily go unnoticed. Harris suggests we attend to the ands (1, 2, 3, 4 "and") in this liminal of spaces where something else happens; vocal phrasing sits there. He would say**,** "if you don't know the ands, you don't know jazz". Tom Anderson noticed this but had a very distinctive style of noticing the ands, as did Milton Erickson and Bradford Keeney, to name only a few. They could all see something else in the room and they knew it, understood it and worked with it from moment to moment. John Shotter may have called it "with-ness thinking" as opposed to "about-ness thinking" (Shotter, 2011). Others may call it the therapeutic alliance (Friedlander et al., 2006) or a liminal space often overlooked. But this "space" or "attitude" is present in most modalities of therapy as well as within the supervisory alliance as discussed in Rønnestad and Lundquist (2009).

Constraint to creativity. There are many moments when we need to step out of the constraints of what our protocols might inform us to do. One of those constraints is the modelling of fidelity, which can have the unfortunate outcome of leading to relational paralysis. Telfener (2016) offers some ideas for moving beyond these points in our practice as supervisors. This involves moving beyond the words we exchange in our supervisory relationship, and encompassing a range of playful, but serious games and techniques to enhance our reflexive positioning. These can be theatrical including movement and body work. Keeney (2014) also highlights how to unlock the constraints and notice our relational edges. This is paying attention to yourself, and the presence you bring to your relationships particularly in supervisory contexts. He proposes that creativity rather than theories, techniques or evidence lead to transformational change, the very process that can unstick the moments of impasse. These acknowledgements are like Naharin's invitation to notice our bones as we dance and their relationship to our skin.

There may always be a queue of informants, people who know, who are willing to offer their expertise on what do next. The manual operator, the model, or working context may be, in itself, part of the problem. Whatever the constraints in a context, it is possible to search for the small space of opportunity—a conversation—since the smallest opportunity can often lead to the biggest changes. Tom Anderson could see these possibilities in breathing out and breathing in (Shotter, 2007). Here, a simple sentence illustrates the opening up of learning and change.

Vignette 2

I am working as a supervisor for a group in a not-for-profit organisation. The supervision is time-limited and retrospective in format. Therefore, the ability to capture moments from small spaces— the "ands"—raises the intensity for the me as the supervisor. How can the learning and development of the group be enhanced in one moment if I dare to capture it? Everyone in the group is a trainee counsellor, although they are all at various stages of their learning and development. One trainee said, "if only I could step into the shoes of the client". The statement came from a theoretical position articulated in a reading for the course she was undertaking. I see this as a gift. I capture and flesh out the idea, attempting to create a self-reflexive context for such a statement. I call this a movement from "skull to skill"—a thinking and doing moment—or from idea to relational framing or simply from inner to outer, but with doing attached to the outer. I am interested in the potential for learning and opening up the possibility for the moment the trainee feels she is stuck and utters the words, "if only I could step into the shoes of the client". I tentatively ask the trainee about doing that, as if, maybe something she has tried with her client therapy work.

The trainee agrees, following the discussion about learning from within the group. The group members agree it is an opportunity. So, I invite them to observe me, thereby giving me the opportunity to receive their feedback and observe the conversation around the dilemma of being stuck. I invite the trainee to put herself in her client's shoes. I talk with the trainee like she is client and present the dilemma to her of her counsellor wishing to be in her shoes to enable her to be useful. What does she think about this idea and can she offer any ideas for this stuck moment in counselling?

The conversation unfolds and lasts for 5–10 minutes. We pause and engage in the delicate process of taking feedback from the observers in what Jones (2003) describes, when quoting Von Foerster (1990), as "a participant actor in the drama of mutual interaction, of the give and take of circularity of Human relations." We hear from everyone and finally the teller of the dilemma, who is now in a different position, multi-layered in the experience and multi-textured in the feedback process. Focusing on the self of the counsellor here may have freed up new possibilities for conversation and action whilst avoiding the blah blah blah (Friere, 2001).

Jones (2003) would affirm this like an old familiar chestnut. The lens of the self of the therapist is key in the orientation towards relational/systemic positioning. Additionally, by asking the questions, what do supervision and the supervisor bring to the construction of the table of stuck-ness, we adopt a relational/systemic positioning. There is always great complexity in these relationships and not shying away from them takes energy, empathy, compassion and critical positioning. This will be clearly evident in a live supervisory moment. Acting in the moment with your trainee team, co-constructing what to do next, is very much like Harris (2012) and his "ands" moment. Jones (2003) also makes it clear that the best use of the relationship with the trainee, consultee, and colleague is the exploration of stuck-ness. It is where learning lies, and it is the edge we sometimes do not reach.

From skull-bound to skill-bound. When creating relational practices, it is key to create and invite our colleagues and trainees to play and see the edges of the practice they wish to develop. However, it takes time to create the context for learning and practice of a relational orientation. The supervisor may be constrained by their own working contexts, like therapy teachers who need to have all the answers at their fingertips, and of course this is not the case, at least for myself. Telfener (2016) has suggested that dealing with stuckness may involve noticing, like Naharin's (2016) position of noticing others, such as boredom, loss of curiosity, and physical and relational fatigue.

The spaces in between. There is possibility that when we notice the spaces in between, opportunity can arise. When this happens, the supervisor can create a context for enabling their supervisees to take what Neden and Burnham (2007) refer to as a relationally reflexive position. A question that invites a stance of relational reflexivity might be, *How are we doing in this moment at this time and in this way?* This is, of course, linked to a self-reflexive position of asking, *How am I doing in this moment at this time in this way?* Additionally, my colleague Kieran Vivian Byrne would add, as we have on many occasions, that we must also consider a complex reflexivity. This we see as resting at the wider contextual levels. It may lead to the question, *How are we doing in this context with its textures and layers?* We can draw upon Pearce's (2005) coordinated management of meaning (CMM) modelling for an extension of our thinking and creating potential options and choices for thinking and unsticking. One example is enhancing our abilities to think contextually and what in CMM terms is the hierarchy model and is one of many choices. This offers us a tool for thinking and is multilayered in this way it invites us to think about speech acts; what is said, by whom, at what time and place make up an episodic moment. This is further layered within a context of relationships, and the consideration of the relationships happening, connected to the past or present and also of the future. This is further connected and woven within a set of scripts, stories, meanings, narratives, micro and grand which connect with each level of the contextual moment. These are nestled within various forces which act to maintain patterns or challenge existing ways of acting and meaning making.

Vignette 3

When working on the second year of our four-year training programme, we frequently ask our participants to work and think about the live work they do. The teaching day on one occasion moved beyond the usual format of the day into what we framed as a practicum, a place of learning—an in-between space—between the practice world of participants and the learning world we create in our course (Hardy & Byrne-Vivian, 2008). However, it is how we scaffold these moments to elicit and create the greatest learning opportunity for all those in the group.

A case/therapeutic dilemma is presented to the group. The dilemma has, as many do, a high degree of complexity. This includes self, relational and complex reflexivity. The participant offering the dilemma is a highly experienced professional as are all of our trainees. The stuck-ness is described, and we tease a relational frame through careful and appreciative inquiry. The actors in the frame emerge through the discussion. There is the practitioner/presenter, the team involved in the work (a multi-professional group), the clients they are working with, as well as others absent or not yet fully connected at the moment. The invitation is made to work with this dilemma and to work in a relationally responsive way. All the group members, approximately 15 people, agree to take part in the unfolding narrative. Some play the team confronting the dilemma. A small group plays the family in therapy and other professionals. There are three distinct episodes that form the practicum: the dilemma offered, responses to it, and reflections about the process observed. This takes a full day and the scaffolding by the teachers takes approximately 2 hours to set up, with the use of one screen, recording and reflections. The afternoon period consists of 3 hours of work that unfold into a complex reflexive experience for the presenter of the dilemma and concludes with an open plenary at the end of the day.

We created the opportunity for the presenter to immerse themselves in the context, almost daring to move into the territory whilst having only the map to go by. This, of course, is an imaginary set of relationships being played out, but one that grows from the presenter's dilemma, descriptions and ongoing contributions, much like a director of a play in a rehearsal.

This event or moment does not happen all of the time, it arises when it arises and when we have the right time and right blend of people who can act into this process. The energy and complexity require constant adjustment to the changing nature of the unfolding narrative within the overall structure of the day. The presenter, on one particular occasion, began to experience a shift from a monologue to dialogue. This was highlighted in the words and language utilised and the shifting nature of the dialogues. It pushed the dilemma and the presenter into creating epilogues of possibility. This transpired after the discussions, thoughts and ideas by and about the practicum experience. This event resonated for many months within the course experience. As I write about it here, it becomes part of the metalogues of such an event, a story about a story being written into another story and so on.

Some of the vignettes offer different positions from which to view stuck-ness. This final vignette highlights the complexity of reflexivity in multiple relationships; it is multi-tasked, multilayered and multi-textured. The presenter is immersed in it, with colleagues co-constructing their own learning moment. This, as Schon (1987) avers, is similar to the relational mud which engulfs the world of practice and is often messy, and we needed to get into the mud with the presenter on this occasion.

The supervisors, like the supervisees, or trainees in this case, also get to take up the learning position. We capture this in the Welsh word DYSGU (pronounced **duss-gee).** It offers the definition of the teacher and learner in one word. I have occupied both positions in the experience of learning and teaching, as well as being a stuck supervisor with a stuck supervisee/colleague/trainee/student. Equally, as a teacher, I am, for the most part, in the learning position as I negotiate with others how we shall learn together in this moment, this day, this session, this lecture, talk, discussion, practicum.

Blah Blah avoidance strategies. Like many relational practices, supervisory relationships carry with them the attention similar to that of providing therapy: ethical decision making, positioning and dis-positioning coalesce around relational being, doing and reflection.

Friere's (2001) position is one which includes the relational responsibility in collaborative processes. This doing without critical reflection can lead to activism. It may be argued that simply observing and instructing does not produce knowledge that contributes to the learning cycle. The transfer of knowledge principle, so endemic in our learning cultures, universities and educational systems, squeeze out the possibilities for transformation and creativity, unlike Keeney's (2014) position of emergent processes which create contexts for learning, change and transformation.

Self of the supervisor. Unlike my self-proclamations, model makers and unified methods and techniques can stifle and create instructive, competence-based technicians. A relational lens offers a multiplicity of ideas and positionings to create contexts for stuck-ness in supervisory relationships to become part of the process of the work that takes place in frames of learning and reflection (Meizerow, 1997).

The social graces Burnham (2008) offers a good example of attending to the self of the supervisor. It invites the promotion of a self-reflexive positioning. This useful nemonic includes: gender, geography, race, religion, age, ability, appearance, class culture, ethnicity and education. It is a nemonic to alert us to the inter-sectionalities we are woven into particularly in supervisory relationships as well as what Jones (2003) sees as important in the supervisory relationships, the attention to the observer position. This enables the supervisor to create with their colleagues in supervision dialogues in which the circular nature of relationships becomes illuminated, and simple but complex questions such as; what contribution do you/I make to the dilemma we have before us or are stuck to or with.

This consideration of social graces is a useful reminder of the inter-sectionalities which are omnipresent and can lead to an extended supervisory repertoire of engaging with, and creating self-reflexive thinking and dialogues. These bring multiple layers of context into focus on themselves[the supervisor], as well as the relationship they are creating with their supervisees. Working within and between contexts is a central idea in the ongoing process of becoming unstuck. It enables us to continue to be creative and construct relational inquiries which can often, and do, lead to changes and transformations.

Ending the Beginnings

This chapter has introduced some established and creative ways of looking at stuck-ness. I have purposefully framed stuck-ness as a competence and as a process of learning which for many does not end in training. For many, it continues to grow in our practice, and we add to our repertoires over time with the ongoing experience and culmination of expertise. Freire (2001) echoes through the chapter as a marker to the tyranny of activism and the impact of Blah Blah Blah.

I have not offered here a specific definition of supervision. Such definitions have been skilfully addressed by previous chapters and writers in the field. Stuck-ness is part of our ongoing relational learning from and with our clients, students and trainees. This chapter makes an invitation to see what we do and how we do it as the artistry of stuck-ness; without it, we may not raise questions, become curious about ourselves, or continue to explore with others how to do this or that. The relationship with ourselves is central to the process and noticing our own bones and skin can remind us of this centrality. I have also suggested we should be attentive to the spaces between, named in this chapter *the ands* (Harris, 2012).

I suggest that we continue to work from the inside out and create relational learning opportunities which I have framed as Skull to Skill. These have been framed as part of the scaffolding and creating of contexts to make strategies for avoiding the blah blah blah (Friere, 2001). Some vignettes from my own practice have hopefully illustrated how being stuck in the middle, requires a repertoire of creativity and the presence of the Supervisor. The invitational stance to relational responsibility is embedded in the scaffolding of the context for learning and transformation. A simple song has encapsulated a moment in time with others, be they clowns and jokers (artists), but useful allays and collaborators in the making of the relationships in supervision. Musical learning and theory from Barry Harris and dance of Ohad Naharin have featured as metaphors of methods from outside our usual therapy domain. Liminal spaces, the ands and the relationship with our skin and bones have been offered as part of the artistic palette upon which we can draw.

Creating repertoires for the artistry of stuck-ness is a collaborative process requiring many of the scaffolding pieces described in this chapter. It is invitational, improvisational and respectful of the relationship and relational frames we engage in a multiplicity of contexts. It is not simply knowledge transfer, but knowledge construction with others. It invites the working towards an embodiment of stuck-ness repertoires, and not the all too frequently espoused positions which may serve to restrain and constrain us.

As layers of creativity form part of the artistry of stuck-ness, it is useful to remember the words of Keeney (2014). He reminds us that creativity calls on the "therapeutic presence of the therapist" and I would suggest, for this chapter, creativity in supervision calls on the *supervisory presence of the supervisor*. Finally, I would like to finish with Bradford Keeney's (2014) pledge to Carl Whittaker, his mentor and colleague (with my contribution in italics), to foster growth of clients with therapists as opposed to the "fix em up" mentality prescribed by simple reductionist models for therapeutic conduct. I should like to pledge to foster growth with supervisees as opposed to the "fix 'em up" mentality of simple reductionist supervisory conduct.

References

Bloom, J. (2016). A Batesonian perspective on qualitative research and complex human systems. In D. Koopmams & D. Stamovlasis (Eds.), *Complex dynamic systems in education* (pp. 23–37). Switzerland: Springer.

Burnham, J., Palma, D., & Whitehouse, L. (2008). Learning as a context for differences and differences as context for learning. *Journal of Family Therapy, 30,* 529–542.

Chen, M., & Noodbond, J. (1999). Unsticking the stuck group system. *Journal of Systemic Therapies, 18*(3), 23–36.

Daniels, H., Cole, M., & Wertsch, J. (Eds). (2007). *The Cambridge companion to Vygotsky.* New York: Cambridge University Press.

Friedlander, M., Escudero, V., & Heatherington, L. (2006). *Therapeutic alliances in couple and family therapy.* Washington: APA.

Friere, P. (2001). *Pedagogy of freedom*. London: Rowman and Littlefield.
Hardy, B., & Byrne-Vivian, K. (2008). With, within and between-creating a learning in practice community multidisciplinary contexts. PEPE, IRISS.org.uk
Harris, B. (2012). *Feeling the ands*, YouTube. February, 2020.
Jones, E. (2003). Working with the self of the therapist in consultation. *Human Systems: the Journal of Consultation and Management, 14*(1), 7–16.
Keeney, B. (2014). *The creative therapist*. London: Routledge.
Laughlin, M. (2000). Teaching creativity in family therapy supervision: Looking through and improvisational lens. *Journal of Systemic Therapies, 19*(3), 55–75.
Mezirow, J. (1997). Transformative learning: Theory to practice. *New Directions for Adult and Continuing Education, 74*(summer), 5–12.
Naharin, O. (2016). *Mr Gaga*, DVD.
Neden, J., & Burnham, J. (2007). Using relational reflexivity as a resource in teaching family therapy. *Journal of Family Therapy, 29*(4), 359–363.
Pearce, W. B. (2005). *The co-ordinated management of meaning*. Retrieved from https://cmminstitute.org/.
Rønnestad, M. H., & Lundquist, K. (2009). *The brief supervisory alliance scale*. Department of Psychology, University of Oslo.
Schon, D. (1987). *The reflective practitioner*. New York: Basic Books.
Shotter, J. (2007). Not to forget Tom Andersen's way of being tom Andersen: The importance of what' just happens' to us. *Human Systems: the Journal of Systemic Consultation and Management, 18*, 15–28.
Shotter, J. (2011). *Getting it: Withness—Thinking and the dialogical in practice*. New York: Hampton Press.
Shurts, M. (2015). Infusing postmodernism into counselling supervision. *Journal of Counsellor Preparation and Supervision, 7*(3) (Art. 5).
Stealers Wheel. (1974). *Stuck in the middle with you*. Released in the UK 1974.
Telfener, U., & Tettamanzi, M. (2016). A bag full of tricks…when therapy feels stuck: How to get over the impasse in difficult situations. *Human Systems: the Journal of Therapy, Consultation and Training, 27*(1), 39–53.

7

'The Difference that Makes a Difference? A Qualitative Study of Cultural Differences and Similarities in Supervision'

Philip Messent and Reenee Singh

Falicov (1998) has defined culture as "those sets of shared world views and adaptive behaviours derived from simultaneous membership in a variety of contexts, such as ecological setting, religious background, nationality and ethnicity, social class, gender-related experience, minority status, occupation, political leaning, migration patterns and stages of acculturation or values derived from belonging to the same generation, partaking of single historical context, or particular ideologies" (p. 336). Culture then is determined by a plethora of different contexts and we will rarely if ever share all these contexts with others, and in this sense "virtually all conversations are cross-cultural" (Gehart, 2016).

P. Messent (✉)
London, UK

R. Singh
London Intercultural Couples Centre, The Child and Family Practice, London, UK

What do we know about what makes for successful cross-cultural supervision? Falicov and Shafransky (2004) suggest that this will involve the development of cross-cultural competency: the "incorporation of self-awareness by both supervisor and supervisee...an interactive encompassing process of the client or family, supervisee-therapist and supervisor, using all of the multiple diversity factors. It entails awareness, knowledge and appreciation of the interactions among the client's, supervisee-therapist's and supervisor's assumptions, values, biases, expectations and world-views, integration and practice of appropriate, relevant and sensitive assessment and intervention strategies and skills, and consideration of the larger milieu of history, society and social-political variables" (p. 125).

This portrays a competency which allows a conversation or process to be created between supervisor and supervisee in which issues of difference can be explored openly, bringing forth a rich discussion involving self-awareness on the part of the supervisor and supervisee, and a cognisance of a host of contextual factors impacting upon client families and shaping how problems are experienced and framed. Hardy (2016) suggests that this will involve supervisors needing to "foster a multicultural relational perspective – a worldview that recognises how the nuances of culture and all of its appendages are contaminants, informants and meaning makers throughout virtually all aspects of our lives" (p. 4).

How do we create contexts in which such rich discussions can take place? A conversational analysis study undertaken by Lawless et al. (2001) gives some clues. This study explored how talk of race, ethnicity and culture (REC) is accomplished within recorded and analysed supervision sessions, finding that opportunities for such talk began in each session with contextual markers such as the ethnicity of the client under discussion. When the supervisor highlighted these markers it led to a richer discussion, not by focussing on the supervisee's knowledge about these areas, but by opening a dialogue about the intersection of REC and other clinical issues. This fits well with Christiansen et al.'s (2011) investigation of the experiences of multicultural supervision of six supervisory candidates on a course and one mentoring supervisor. They agreed that all instances of multicultural supervision discussed were unplanned, occurring spontaneously, and arising out of the content of therapy or supervision.

Sohelian et al.'s (2014) study further investigated supervisees' perceived experiences of multicultural competence in supervision by analysing the experience of 102 supervisees. Multiculturally competent supervisors were seen as facilitating the exploration of specific cultural issues, discussing culturally appropriate therapeutic interventions and skills, facilitating supervisee self-awareness within the supervision session, and challenging and encouraging cultural openness in supervisees' understandings of cultural issues.

There is an emphasis throughout the literature (e.g. Chenfeng, 2016; Falicov & Shafranske, 2004; Hardy, 2016; Pendry, 2012, 2017; Watson, 2016) that it is the responsibility of the supervisor to create opportunities for such discussions, lest supervisees feel that they are inappropriate or not relevant. There is also broad agreement about the need to create the right atmosphere for such discussions, embracing a stance of compassion (Falicov & Shafranske, op. cit., Hardy, op. cit.,) and a 'community of safety' (Chenfeng, op. cit.), in which supervisees can explore their own identity without 'the threat of ever feeling one-down or unvalued'.

Creating such an atmosphere will be helped by openness and self-reflexivity on the part of the supervisor, and an acknowledgement of any 'missteps'; Hardy (op. cit.) suggests we must seek to turn these into 'steady steps', demonstrating a willingness to make mistakes and to be vulnerable, 'staying connected', and to talk about what happened. I (PM) have written elsewhere (Messent, 2017) about how my learning in supervising across difference has often occurred when something has 'felt wrong' to me—either a supervisee has demonstrated some degree of discomfort, or I have felt some sense of unease. It has not always been possible to unravel and make sense of such discomfort in the moment and has required a willingness on my part to be open about my contribution to these moments, for mutual learning to occur. As Sohelian et al. (op. cit.) suggest, there is 'struggle' involved in this process: all of the case examples focussed on by the 7 participants involved in this study spoke of negative emotional reactions being present (i.e. discomfort, anxiety, and anger). Gehart (op. cit.) suggests that cross-cultural supervision at such moments will require 'relational responsibility' in which we seek to understand the good behind the others' actions.

Implicit in much of the above is a need to address the impact of power relationships and privilege upon relationships (Hardy, op. cit.), which will begin with the supervisory relationship, then widen to include client families and the systems surrounding them. There will also be a need to acknowledge discrimination, racism and their impacts (Falicov & Shafranske, op. cit.). Watson (op. cit.) suggests that, race is a particularly critical context for such inquiry, requiring supervisors and therapists to grapple with their racial selves as well as that of their clients. They note that this is within a general duty of supervisors to help supervisees understand their multiple contexts and identities in order that they recognize and appreciate their clients' multiple contexts and identities.

In the study reported in this chapter, we interviewed our supervisees about their experiences of having supervisors of the same or different cultures. We were interested in further developing our understanding of what these experiences were like, and any lessons emerging about how supervision across differences in culture can go well. PM interviewed a supervisee of African Ghanaian heritage working in the UK (M), and a group of Bangladeshi supervisees working in Dhaka, Bangladesh—in this case adding a further complexity of this supervision being across international boundaries. RS interviewed a supervision group that comprised two Iranian counsellors (S1 and S2) working with Iranian Farsi speaking clients and their culturally and linguistically matched supervisor, S. She had supervised the two counsellors in their clinical practice and had been S's doctoral research supervisor. The supervisees were hence able to reflect on their experiences both of culturally matched supervision and intercultural supervision. S, who is highly experienced, drew on her vast experience, as both supervisee and supervisor in varied settings, making for a particularly rich conversation between RS and the supervision group.

Interviews and Analysis

We devised an interview protocol which drew upon the supervisees' experiences of culturally matched and intercultural supervision (see Appendix for the interview protocol). The interviews were recorded, transcribed and analysed using the qualitative method of Thematic Analysis. Braun and Clarke (2006) define thematic analysis as: "a method for identifying, analyzing and reporting patterns within data" (p. 79). Within a range of qualitative methods, thematic analysis was chosen as it was considered the simplest and least 'fussy'. We were aware of the complexity of the research design and wanted a simple clustering of themes that would allow the participants' voices, across all three sets of data, to speak for themselves.

In analysing the transcribed interviews, we deployed a line by line analysis, then clustered together the emerging themes into higher order constituent themes and superordinate themes. We used verbatim quotations from the participants to present the findings in a narrative form.

Themes from Iranian Supervision Group

The interviews seemed to cluster into two overarching themes, which I (RS) have named 'Closeness/distance in intercultural/intracultural[1] supervision' and 'Complexity of intercultural therapy/supervision' (See Appendix for tables of themes). Because of the constraints of space, it is not possible to explore each sub-theme in detail, but I will touch on the key constituent themes, accompanied by verbatim quotations from the participants.

---

[1]The terms intercultural and intracultural supervision will be used in this analysis to refer to supervision across cultural difference (often referred to in the literature as 'cross-cultural') and supervision that is provided within culture.

Theme 1: Closeness/Distance in Intercultural/Intracultural Supervision

The first theme relates to the idea of the 'difference that makes the difference' (Bateson, 2000). How experience near or experience far should supervision be in order for it to be most useful? The theme also encompasses the fit between supervisor and supervisee in intracultural or culturally matched supervision. The constituent themes are 'homeness', language, curiosity and choice.

The first constituent theme that emerged from the material was '**homeness**', a term I have borrowed from Papadopoulous (2017) to denote feeling 'at home', comfortable or familiar. In describing her experiences of supervising those from a similar cultural background, S explains:

> ....It does feel like home. It doesn't even feel like supervision. If feels like a conversation where they say 'so and so said this' and we all look at each other and go 'ah ha' (laughter). It's just, we just get it, it really is a conversation... and that felt very homely.

This experience of 'homeness' seems to come from familiarity with the context as well as the content; a sense of not having to explain oneself and of feeling understood. Supervisee 1 captures this feeling in her words:

> I don't need to explain when I say something....she gets the context.... however, if I speak with a supervisor from a different culture, they might say 'oh my God, that's horrible'. But they actually haven't seen the war. They haven't seen how, what the revolutionary guard can do to you when they get your car and stop your car and they, you know question you....

However, this shared understanding may be experienced as not professional enough or 'too cosy':

> Supervisee 2: 'However, sometimes um, sometimes I feel because of our culture we are very friendly we sort of like, we get into the mood that ok, just relax. This is fine. Sometimes I feel like we are, I feel that we lost that content of this is a professional gathering are we are here to just

sort of explore what is going on with the therapy in a client or myself. Sometimes I feel I might not get what I need.

This seems to be the both/and nature of culturally matched supervision—the sense of comfort, familiarity or 'homeness' is experienced by the supervisees as facilitating understanding, yet sometimes may feel too close to perturb their understanding of their clients' experiences.

Language. Part of the comfort of culturally matched supervision appears to come from the shared use of language. As Supervisee 1 expounds,

> It's different because when we talk in your mother tongue and it's, I mean it's there, it's just that you don't have to think about it. But when you are speaking in another language, a second language, sometimes you can't find the words. And sometimes you find it difficult even when you are fluent in that language, sometimes you can't find what you want to say in the most appropriate, for example, word or phrase or even sentence. Although you are used to that language, but it's always there is a barrier there....

The linguistically matched supervisor appears to grasp not just the meaning of the language, but also the nuances and the slang:

> Supervisee 2: The language is sort of like allowing us to be very present in the moment and sort of acknowledging – Ok, (the supervisor, S). will know this slang...because with our culture, for sure Persian culture, when we speak, we don't speak directly. It's everything is indirectly through slang and through phrases....

Speaking in the same language appears to be even more important when talking about emotions:

> Supervisee 1; When I work with my clients who speak Farsi, even those clients who have been raised here...when they want to talk about emotions and deeper feelings they go into Farsi immediately...they use both languages, but deeper emotions they just start speaking Farsi.

Hence, it can help to speak to a linguistically matched supervisor about the strong emotions that the clients, their therapists, and the supervisees can only express in their mother tongue. In the words of Supervisee 2:

> …If I want to express really my emotion and my difficulties or my client's difficulties, maybe it's about, it is some language barrier for me to express. Maybe the (cross cultural) supervisor would not understand. I think mainly it's just the language that will create a feeling for me… maybe the supervisor will miss something there or did I really express myself there?

Hence, a supervisor from a different cultural and linguistic background may not understand and the meaning of what the supervisee is attempting to explain, may get 'lost in translation.' However, in keeping with Burck's (2005) seminal research, sometimes English can provide a helpful distance in which strong emotions, such as anger can be expressed:

> Supervisee 1: When I am angry, I just switch to English. I think it was the first year when I arrived in this country in 1994 I think, and I was talking on the phone. My English was very, very weak then and I was trying and struggling to talk to this person on the phone from one of these companies and I got angry. Suddenly I switched into English and then it's fluent. And I couldn't understand it (laughs). Then when I hung up I said 'what happened?' I know all this English? It was very interesting.

Thus, speaking to a supervisor from a different cultural and linguistic background could open up a different linguistic space, which could allow a range of emotions not possible in one's mother tongue.

Curiosity. Whether supervision is intercultural or intracultural, the supervisor's curiosity about the supervisee's clinical practice seems to be an important aspect of supervision. However, it is easy, in either clinical practice or supervision for the therapist/supervisor from the same cultural background to **make assumptions** and **lose curiosity**:

> S: I remember I was working with an Iranian client once as a therapist who came from the south of Iran, like real South, almost border to Iraq.

And I said to him, 'oh yeah, you know, I understand because we're from the same culture.' He said, 'No, no we're not. We're completely different cultures because I'm from the south of Iraq.' And he taught me a lot. They have tribal life, you know. They're all tribes. And he said we are more Arab than Iranian. We eat Arabic, we speak Arabic….so it's assuming that you know when you don't.

However, the intercultural supervisor might also make assumptions:

Supervisee 2: …The danger is you perceive something in your own way and you think this is what is happening, when it is not. You need to check.

Judgemental. Sometimes, an intimate knowledge of the culture can lead to the supervisor from the same background being judgemental:

Supervisee 2: It was a typical Persian man, you know, very traditional and very controlling. Um, and the wife was sort of like still stayed in the situation. It wasn't very abusive, but the man was very, very traditional…and when I presented the case, the group's idea was she has to get rid of him, you know kick him out…. because of the background, because we know how Persian men can be, we are already judging that guy. If it was a non-Persian supervisor right away might have asked something different… the judgement doesn't allow us to look at the depth of the issue.

Thus, being deeply embedded in a culture might lead to a supervisor from the same or a similar cultural background to make assumptions and judgements.

To summarize, a supervisor from a similar cultural background may embody 'homeness'; the linguistic fit might be helpful but at the same time, this closeness may lead to the supervisor losing curiosity. So how close or distant should supervision be in order for it to be most helpful? This is explored through the fourth subtheme, of choice.

Choice. Although S, the supervisor said that she would seek out a supervisor from the same cultural background if she had a choice, Supervisee 1 said that the cultural background was not as important as 'feeling comfortable'. Supervisee 2 thought that it was important to have experiences of both intercultural and culturally matched supervision:

> And I think it's important to acknowledge how this culture is helping trauma, for instance, complex trauma, and how we as Persians are dealing with that trauma and having that experience and acknowledging what is the difference...the combination of both I think will be more beneficial for the client and the therapist to have an experience of both.

Further, she wondered whether the choice of whether to have an intercultural supervisor or someone from a similar background was dependent on how assimilated into the host culture the supervisee is. For a supervisee who is more Iranian, an Iranian Farsi speaking supervisor may be more suitable whereas a supervisor from a different cultural background may be a better fit for a supervisee who was more open to "experiencing and learning new things".

Theme 2: Complexity of Intercultural Therapy/Supervision

Reflecting on their experiences of intercultural and culturally matched supervision, S and both supervisees acknowledged the complexity of this work.

'No race' talk. Consistent with the literature (see, e.g., Pendry, 2012) one of the difficulties is in bringing up issues of race within a supervisory group. Describing her experiences of being supervised by a French, Lacanian supervisor, S says:

> But what was really odd...was that in those days we never spoke about race. So I would be working with all these like African families and Algerian families and not once would we talk about culture or race. And I always remember coming out thinking there's something missing and I didn't get what I wanted there. There's something missing....

In another supervision group where she was the supervisor, she had a similar difficulty in addressing race, for fear of causing offence to her black supervisee. She concludes that it comprises 'taking a relational risk to talk about racism'. When the supervisor does not directly address issues of 'race' and racism, it is incumbent upon the supervisee from a minority ethnic background to bring this up. This can feel tokenistic, or as if it is the black and minority ethnic supervisee's responsibility to speak on behalf of 'race' and culture:

> S: There is no culture of culture…it really is kind of like, you know, thinking theoretically about families but not thinking about their culture, about their race. So we're (naming two black colleagues) the ones who are bringing in the culture all the time and it's a bit uncomfortable a lot of the time….

Norm is different in different cultures. Another sub-theme relating to the complexity of intercultural supervision is that the 'norm is different in different cultures'. 'The family', parenting and gendered roles are constructed differently in different cultures and in intercultural supervision, these norms may be misunderstood.

> S1 Years ago I was an interpreter for a counsellor working for an Afghan family. Apparently in Afghan families, mothers use older girls to look after the younger ones and help around the house, do chores and all these things. And when the counsellor had talked to the child, to the girl, and she was accusing the mother of not loving her child….and I know, of course, one of the most important things for Afghani women is motherhood and being a good mother.

In this example, the **intersection** between gender and culture emerged, as well as the differences between a white, western feminist position as compared to a position where there is a recognition from the therapist/supervisor that oppression and gendered roles have different meanings in different cultures. Effective supervision was seen as a process of joining across cultural differences and being able to name difference and challenge cultural assumptions.

To conclude, the two interrelated themes of Closeness/Distance in culturally matched supervision and the complexity of intercultural practice/supervision emerged in the interviews with my Iranian, Farsi speaking participants. The findings call for a 'both-and' position, recognizing the need both for supervision from a culturally and linguistically matched supervisor as well as those from other cultural backgrounds, who are able to be genuinely curious and willing to talk about issues of 'race' and racism.

Themes from Interview with M

I (PM) named four overarching themes emerged from my interview with a supervisee of African Ghanaian heritage as: 'context makes a difference', 'experience and theoretical orientation', 'sharing a culture makes communication easier' and 'aspects of the supervisory process which make for good intracultural supervision'.

Theme 1: Context Makes a Difference

Much of the supervision literature refers to supervision within training courses, but this does not do justice to the range of different contexts in which supervision takes place, and the way that context changes the nature of the supervisory relationship and the kind of conversations that take place. These too can be seen as differences in 'culture': a culture of assessment in a training course places limits on ease of communication, while a supervisor outside an organization can offer a wider perspective than one within it.
   Part of training course v outside training course.

> The main difference for me is knowing that I'm being assessed. So it doesn't feel as relaxed... I'm always thinking that I have to say the right thing.

For M, the context of independent supervision allowed her more of a sense of relaxation, and less of a sense of having to get things right.
   Internal/managerial v external/independent.
   Supervisors internal to organizations, who may also be in a position of line-managers (the supervision which many in public service

contexts rely upon) may be involved in the case under discussion in a way which places limits upon their perspective, and the possibility of offering something helpful.

> the best thing about it (i.e. external supervision) is having another, a third eye, and if you've got someone who is 'in it' and going through it with you and working with the same client group, sometimes it is difficult for them to really stand back

Theme 2: Experience and Theoretical Orientation

How supervision goes will also be determined by the level of experience and training of the supervisor and the theoretical fit with the supervisee. M recounted an unsatisfactory experience of an untrained supervisor who had not been helpful, and another where a supervisor brought a medical focus to discussions which did not fit well with her therapeutic intentions. This too can amount to a cultural difference in underlying beliefs about the purpose and orientation of the work.
Level of training and experience of supervisor.

> I think that because she was not a trained supervisor there were times when she wasn't as helpful as I needed her to be.

Supervisors provided internally by organizations may have little or no formal training in supervision, which is likely to place limits upon their helpfulness.
Differences in theoretical orientation.
Supervisors provided internally may also have different ways of understanding the nature of difficulties and their possible resolution which fit poorly with supervisees, for example in this example of one of M's supervisors' ideas about the underlying medical nature of problems under discussion:

> it was quite medicalised as well… that doesn't really fit for me.

Theme 3: Sharing a Culture Makes Communication Easier

Similarities across culture make for easier communication, with less need to explain.
This seemed to fit closely with the theme of 'homeness' in the Iranian group described above associated here for M with shared gender and/or cultural/social/locational backgrounds.

> as women, not only in terms of race but also in terms of gender we have a certain language that we speak, so that there were certain things that I felt that I did not have to explain

This shared sense of similarity of backgrounds may extend also to clients, allowing for an ease in communication grounded on shared lived experience and mutual understanding:

> I was working in an environment in which there were lots of kids from different cultural backgrounds …and there was something similar in my background and her background which made it easier for us to have those conversations…to talk about those kids.

Need to explain more (and take care of) white supervisors.
In complete contrast to this, more needs to be explained to white supervisors: for example, where racism has been an aspect of a case under discussion with me (PM), M had felt that (far from building on shared experiences) she had to take extra care to make clear that I am not being also described as racist:

> Sometimes I have thought that I've had to explain that … I'm not talking about you, I'm talking about other white people that behave in that way.

Theme 4: Aspects of the Supervisory Process Which Make for Good Intracultural Supervision

A number of practices that contributed towards the supervisory process going well fitted well with systemic methodology: regular review to ensure feedback is heard and responded to; maintaining curiosity to avoid making assumptions, and maintaining an interest in and responding to the experience of the individual supervisee rather than focussing only on content.

Talking about/reviewing the process of supervision.
M described how a new systemic supervisor had reviewed with her how the supervisory process was going, after a period in which she had felt that things had not been going well, and made changes accordingly:

> I was then working psychodynamically and I really struggled with it (systemic supervision)... I found that once we'd sat down and talked about it, he tried to not only adapt his style...but also he was very supportive

Listening and curiosity of supervisor and not making assumptions.
M stressed the importance of supervisors not making assumptions, asking questions from a position of curiosity, and really listening:

> In supervision with you, you are always curious and you ask me questions, and you want to know. And that means to me that you are listening, and that you are not making assumptions and you are wanting to be helpful, and I find that really helpful.

Supervisor being interested in supervisee's experience.
Systemic supervision has as its focus the client, their context and the supervisee's experience: it is this *interaction* that is discussed. M described two examples of times when her supervisor's focus had been (unhelpfully) exclusively upon case material, rather than including also something of her own experience during the work that had been undertaken:

So, where supervision hasn't worked is where that hasn't happened.... I've had two experiences of that, one was with a male, one was with a woman. And actually, the woman was black, so it wasn't about the racial thing, ... it felt as though she was doing everything by the book, and not really interested in what was going on for me... She was only interested in the cases...Let's talk about this case, this child, what was going on with the child. But not what was going on for me or what my experience was.

To conclude, four themes emerging from this interview regarding a number of different supervision experiences were: the significance of the context within which supervision takes place; the level of experience and training of the supervisor and the theoretical fit with the supervisee; the way in which a shared culture between supervisor and supervisee eases communication between them; and the way in obstacles to communication across cultural difference can be overcome.

Themes from Supervision Across Region Interview

Four similar overarching themes emerged from my (PM) interview with the group of Bangladeshi supervisees: 'language difference as a barrier and ways that this is mitigated'; 'understanding is facilitated by the systemic model'; 'shared experience creates understanding'; and 'trust in the effectiveness of the model and of the competence of the supervisor'.

Theme 1: Language Difference as Barrier and Ways that This Is Mitigated

While the difference in first language between supervisees and supervisor was seen as an obstacle to ease of understanding and communication (as with the Iranian group above), group members spoke of ways in which such difficulties could be overcome.

In understanding supervisor, and in spontaneity of expression.
Supervisees spoke of how a supervisor who could speak Bangla would have made for easier and more spontaneous communication.

> A supervisor from the same language and culture would be helpful for our group, as it will facilitate communication.
>
> **Usefulness though of written summaries of supervision meetings in overcoming this barrier.** Supervisees spoke of the helpfulness of the supervisor producing a written summary of key learning points following each supervision meeting. What may have been missed or only partially understood during the meeting, could be thus revisited in a written form, allowing for reflection at the supervisee's own pace.
>
> This is one of the most productive parts'

Such difficulties were also mitigated by the fact that all other texts and constructs learnt as part of these supervisees' original psychology training had been in English, so supervisees would have to 'double translate' if teaching/supervision were to be in Bangla. They were used to learning in English and this fitted with the language of their previous training.

Theme 2: Understanding Facilitated by Systemic Model

As with M, aspects of the systemic method helped to ensure that culture was seen by supervisees as included and understood: the way that culture is routinely addressed as part of all case and theoretical discussion, the way that curiosity, self-reflexivity and respect is maintained, a non-judgemental attitude, and care taken in connecting with models of therapy already in use.

Overarching Systemic method as a resource.
The lens provided by the systemic model was seen as always inclusive of culture, ensuring that there was no 'gap' in understanding between the supervisor and the supervisees:

> my experience is..you fit everything into your systemic concept..you interpret in systemic concepts so I don't feel any gap.

> Though you are from a different culture you understand and make sense of all of our cultural content and conflict.

Use of curiosity, self-reflexivity and respect.
Supervisees saw their supervisor as curious, self-aware and respectful towards their culture, and careful not to make suggestions which might run counter to cultural norms:

> I find my supervisor is curious about our culture, language, tradition, family script, and is aware about his own..He always tries to control his background and is respectful about Bangladeshi culture
>
> My supervisor was very serious about respect for culture, and never provided anything that might go against our norms..

Acceptance and a non-judgmental attitude.
Supervisees new to the systemic model valued an opportunity to present work without fear of critical judgement, helped by the position taken by the supervisor of valuing the efforts being made by supervisees to introduce this new model of practice:

> We feel free to share whatever we did, right or wrong..

Systemic model inclusive of existing orientation (CBT).
The supervisees' existing training as clinical psychologists drew principally on the cognitive behavioural approach and there had at the start of their training been some misgivings expressed as to whether this might interfere with, or disrupt this approach to their work. Such misgivings were now felt to have been unnecessary, with systemic supervision being seen as sympathetic to and enhancing this approach:

> I thought that SFT would interfere but I think it has added another powerful sense, like my eyes and ears..
>
> SFT increases our skill and we can apply CBT more effectively.

Theme 3: Shared Experience Creates Understanding

Some experience of one another's country and culture was seen as helpful in aiding mutual understanding, as well as a sense that problems and people's feelings were not significantly different in our two countries. Cultural stereotypes about Western culture (which may have otherwise been an obstacle to understanding) were overcome through experience.
Problems similar across cultures.
Some supervisees had experience of working in the UK and saw problems experienced, feelings and family responses as similar:

> I found psychiatric cases in the UK and in Bangladesh are very similar'
> 'In a family crisis there will be many similarities.. Language is different but feelings are the same..

Cultural understanding of supervisor through earlier visits/trainings helpful.
Similarly, the supervisor's previous visits to the country (to deliver training) were seen as valuable in giving some understanding of the culture:

> ..because you came here in Bangladesh, you have a fair idea of the culture

Prejudices about cultural difference of supervisor overcome.
Supervisees' assumptions about cultural differences (which may have been an obstacle to understanding) had been changed through the process of the developing supervisory relationship:

> I had a schema that Western people were .. too much work-focussed (but) ..I have found empathy from you..

Theme 4: Trust in the Effectiveness of the Model and of the Competence of the Supervisor Helpful

Trust and confidence in supervision in this model had been strengthened by knowledge of his accreditation as a supervisor and by his perceived knowledge of the model:
The supervisor's qualifications and perceived competence.

> When you supervise me I know I am getting supervision from an accredited supervisor
>
> You know your subject very well.. so when you supervise, we feel confidence..

The way that systemic explanations/hypotheses fitted well for client families under discussion, and by the impact of supervised work on those families.

Trust and confidence in the model had been further strengthened through the way that its explanations were found to have fitted for client families that were discussed in supervision, and then by its perceived impact upon these families, and the way they were left feeling 'light', as demonstrated by their feedback:

> I find your explanation fits well.. Later on with clients I see that they work very well'
>
> My client feedback has been increased tremendously after having this knowledge, the Systemic Family Therapy (SFT)..The beauty of SFT is that it makes the client feel light, not heavy.

Discussion and Key Learning Points for Supervisors

In the discussion that follows, key learning points emerging from this process will be in bold. There are some striking similarities between themes emerging from these three interviews, as well as some differences. Some important contextual differences may account for some differences in themes emerging, for example in the interview with M, difference in language was not an issue, with both supervisor and supervisee having English as a first language. With the Bangladeshi group, participants had little or no experience of supervision from within their culture and in their first language to compare with the supervision they had received in English, which may account for the lack of equivalent talk about the sense of comfort and 'Homeness' described so vividly by the Iranian group. They have had to get used to using English in academic work as all education at degree level and above is delivered in English and papers and professional papers and training material is also in English, hence as one supervisee said, if supervision were to be in Bangla, they would need to translate back to English to connect it to the language that has been relied upon for much of their professional training. M's descriptions of not having to explain things to supervisors and co-supervisees of similar intersecting cultures however fitted well with this sense of a shared 'Homeness'.

There sometimes appears to be very little that a supervisor from a different cultural background can do to understand the context in which the supervisees and their clients' lives are embedded. I (RS) was humbled by the knowledge that, unlike S, I would never fully comprehend the embodied experiences of torture and political trauma. I realized that the **gaps in my understanding could only be met by a willingness to respect, witness and stay with the supervisees' pain,** felt on behalf of their clients.

Both groups experienced language difference as an obstacle to ease of communication, though there was little of the more nuanced discussion during the interview with the Bangladeshi group about how different languages fitted better for communicating about emotional states. One way of easing these difficulties mentioned by one supervisee was the supervisor **providing a written summary** after each session, so that key points could be gone over again after the supervision meeting. Another supervisory practice that has proven helpful with this group also mentioned in the discussion has been pausing for a conversation in Bangla between the supervision group, where one member of the group has felt unclear about what is being communicated in English. In systemic training delivered by PM and colleagues to this group (which led to the practice being supervised in this group) the need to find an ease in Bangla in applying the model has been foregrounded throughout, with training sessions similarly paused at times to ensure understanding, and regular opportunities for group members to discuss in Bangla the material taught and its fit with Bangladeshi culture and working contexts (Fredman et al., 2018).

Sharing a culture for both the Iranian group and for M contributed to making communication easier; both spoke of the greater comfort and ease in mutual understanding, both referring also to the way in which intersections between different shared cultures such as gender, race and social background meant less need for laboured explanations. Cultural similarity did not in itself however guarantee such shared understanding: M describes how one Black supervisor has been preoccupied unhelpfully with case content as opposed to M's experience. In both interviews, there was reference also to the way that the shared perspective that came from a shared culture could come at a cost, leading to assumptions and a lack of curiosity on the part of the culturally matched supervisor (mentioned by S), and a lack of the distance necessary for the supervisor to offer a helpfully different perspective (M).

The complexities involved in discussions about racial differences feature for both S and for M. S reports on a situation where it has been left to Black supervisees to raise such issues as they occur in the work described; another situation where she has felt a lack with her supervisor failing to address this; and a third situation where she has felt uncomfortable as a supervisor raising this issue for fear of causing offence to a black supervisee. M speaks about how with other Black supervisees and Black supervisors, especially where gender also is shared, that because of a 'certain language' this is shared (in part also because of a shared social background), there are things that don't have to be explained. With a White supervisor however she feels a need to let him know that he is not implicated, that when talking about racism, she is talking about 'other' white people and not him.

I (PM) learnt from this that despite a supervisory relationship of several years in which I had aimed to take supervisory responsibility for ensuring that the impacts of race and racism were included in our discussions, M was feeling a need to make clear that she did not see me as being involved in such racism, in this way protecting my feelings. I have realized therefore **a need for white supervisors to explicitly acknowledge our own involvement in privilege, discrimination and racism through our membership of an inherently racist society, signalling a willingness to take responsibility for such involvement, and to be challenged where we are failing to see this, rejecting a defensiveness born from what Diangelo (2018) has described as 'white fragility'.** Such a stance will necessitate not leaving it to our black supervisees to be the ones to raise issues of race as these may emerge in the work, and acknowledging our own limited perspectives, and need to learn about experiences that we do not share.

There are also a number of commonalities between the themes arising from the interviews regarding the usefulness of the systemic methodology in navigating the territory of both intracultural and intercultural supervision. **Maintaining curiosity** featured in all the interviews as an important factor: helping therapists or supervisors from the same cultural background to avoid making assumptions: M saw her intercultural supervisor's curiosity as linked to 'listening' and not making assumptions; one of the Bangladeshi group linked this to the intercultural supervisor's self-reflexivity and respect for their culture.

Other important systemic methods and stances were also seen as helpful: the Bangladeshi group spoke of appreciating their supervisor's **acceptance and a non-judgmental attitude. Avoiding contradicting existing models** was also important: for M her supervisor had 'adapted his style' to fit with her (at that stage) preferred psychodynamic model, for the Bangladeshi group the systemic approach had added to their previous CBT approach, rather than 'interfering' with it. Similarly, the Iranian supervisees were trained in psychodynamic and humanistic integrative models, respectively, and the supervisory space provided a synthesis of systemic ideas with their existing knowledge. Such alternative models are also like a culture that supervisors may share, forming a web of intersecting beliefs about what is important in the work.

The Bangladeshi group also saw their supervisor as **including culture in case discussions** so that cultural content and conflict is 'made sense of', so that there is no 'gap' in understanding. In this supervision context across national borders, culture is an ever-present 'contextual marker', triggering routinely the sort of rich discussions noted by Lawless, Gale and Bacigalupe (op cit).

An openness to reviewing the supervisory process, accepting feedback about where supervision has not been helpful is also demonstrated as important in M's account of how after a discussion with her supervisor, he had modified his style and this had made the supervision more helpful. Such an openness accords with the UK Association of Family Therapy's supervision 'Information Sheet' (2018) with its recommendation for supervisors to 'be open to discussion, co-creation of ideas and constructive feedback', and 'to actively consider issues of power and difference, for example in relation to gender, race, culture, class, age, economic status, disability, sexual orientation, religion and spirituality'.

It is important to note that the interviews were carried out before the outbreak of COVID-19, and before the tragic murder of George Floyd. In a sense, our research—across these three different supervisory experiences located in three different cultural contexts—could be seen as prescient in highlighting the significance of such difference. We wondered though, how our conversations might have been different and what themes may have emerged if the interviews had taken place later in the year, and how these two, unprecedented global events would have shaped our conversations about racial and cultural similarities and differences within supervisory processes.

Appendix

Interview Protocol

Supervisees

1. Please explain a bit about the context of your clinical practice (Prompts—what kinds of clients do you work with?)
2. What kind of arrangements for supervision have you made, or have been made for you? Could you tell me a bit about the contexts for supervision? (Prompt—Is the supervision part of a training context?)

3. What prompted you to choose a supervisor from a similar/different cultural background? (if you made this choice)
4. In what way, would you say, have your experiences of cross-cultural supervision been different from your experiences of supervision with a culturally matched supervisor? (where you have had experiences of both)
5. What do you think your supervisor from a similar cultural background (where you have had this experience) most understood and appreciated about you and your clients?
6. What do you think your supervisor from a different cultural background (where you have had this experience) least understood and appreciated about you and your clients' experience?
7. Is there anything else you think I should have asked you about your experiences of supervision from someone who is similar or different from you in cultural background?

Supervisors

1. Please tell me something about your supervisory experiences—the history, the kinds of clients you have supervised, and the contexts of supervision (training or otherwise)
2. In what way do you think supervising clients from the same/a similar cultural background to you can be a constraint, and in what ways do you think it can be an advantage?
3. What ways have you found to be most successful in working well together across differences in culture in supervision?
4. Is there anything else you would like to tell me/you think I should have asked you about your experiences?

Themes from Interview with Iranian Group

Closeness/Distance in Intercultural/Intracultural Supervision	Complexity of intercultural therapy/supervision
Homeness	'No race' talk
Language	Intersections of gender, class, religion and culture
Curiosity	'The norm' different in different cultures
Choice	Success comes from joining/challenging
	Constant interplay between similarity and difference
	Tokenism-speaking on behalf of culture
	Cultural similarities are a higher context marker than religious differences

Constituent Themes for 'Closeness/Distance'

7 'The Difference that Makes ...   145

Homeness	Language	Curiosity	Choice
Familiarity	Mother tongue 'natural'	Losing curiosity	Would choose a supervisor from the same cultural background if possible
Comfortable	Don't have to think in mother tongue	Making assumptions	Having to seek cultural consultation outside supervision
'Getting it'/not getting it	Linguistic understanding of idiom	Judgemental	Both/and—important to have experiences of both intercultural and intracultural supervision.
Being understood—no need to explain	Emotions expressed easily in mother tongue	Possibilities to challenge intracultural/intercultural supervisor	The fit between the supervisor and supervisee depends on supervisee's assimilation to the dominant culture.
Understanding context of torture and trauma	Language as a barrier		
Explanation important	English provides the distance in which to express strong emotions like anger		
Too cosy!	Too emotional/too angry		
Losing the edge	Language allows us to be present 'in the moment'.		

(continued)

Homeness	Language	Curiosity	Choice
Not professional enough	What gets lost in translation		
Hitting a wall			
Visceral and embodied responses			
Empathy			

Themes from Interview with M

Context makes a difference	Experience and theoretical orientation	Sharing culture makes communication easier	What makes for good cross-cultural supervision
Part of training course vs outside training course	Level of training and experience of supervisor	Similarities across gender, race, 'backgrounds' and intersections between these	Talking about/reviewing the process of supervision
Internal/managerial vs external/independent	Differences in theoretical orientation	Need to explain more, and look after white supervisor when discussing racism	Listening and curiosity of supervisor and not making assumptions Supervisor being interested in supervisee's experience

Themes from Interview with Bangladeshi Group

Language difference as barrier and ways that this mitigated	Cultural difference not an obstacle as understanding facilitated by systemic model	Other reasons why cultural difference not an obstacle	Trust in the effectiveness of the model and of the competence of the supervisor
In understanding supervisor, and in spontaneity of expression	Systemic method as a resource	Problems similar across cultures	The supervisor's qualifications and perceived competence
Usefulness though of written summaries	Use of curiosity, self-reflexivity and respect	Cultural understanding of supervisor	Fit of systemic explanations and impact of work on clients

(continued)

(continued)			
Language difference as barrier and ways that this mitigated	Cultural difference not an obstacle as understanding facilitated by systemic model	Other reasons why cultural difference not an obstacle	Trust in the effectiveness of the model and of the competence of the supervisor
Mitigated also by fact that all other texts and constructs are in English	Acceptance and a non-judgemental attitude	Prejudices about cultural difference of supervisor overcome	
	Fit of systemic model with existing orientation		

References

Association of Family Therapy. (2018). *AFT supervision information sheet.* https://www.aft.org.uk/SpringboardWebApp/userfiles/aft/file/Information%20Sheets/Supervision%20Information%20Sheet%20May%202018.pdf. Accessed 27 August 2020.

Bateson, G. (2000). *Steps to an ecology of mind: Collected essays in anthropology, psychiatry, evolution and epistemology.* The University of Chicago Press.

Braun, V., & Clarke, V. (2006). Using thematic analysis in Psychology. *Journal of Qualitative Research in Psychology, 3*(2), 77–101.

Burck, C. (2005). *Multilingual living.* Palgrave.

ChenFeng, J. L. (2016). From invisibility to embrace: Promoting culturally sensitive practices in supervision. In K. V. Hardy & T. Bobes (Eds.), *Culturally sensitive supervision and training: Diverse perspectives and practical applications.* Routledge.

Christiansen, A. T., Thomas, V., Kafescioglu, N., Karakurt, G., Lowe, W., Smith, W., & Wittneborn, A. (2011). Multicultural supervision: Lessons learned about an ongoing struggle. *Journal of Marital and Family Therapy, 37* (1), 109–119.

Diangelo, R. (2018). *White fragility: Why it's so hard for White people to talk about racism*. Beacon Press.

Falicov, C. J. (1998). *The Guilford family therapy series. Latino families in therapy: A guide to multicultural practice*. Guilford Press.

Falicov, C. J., & Shafranske, E. P. (2004). *Clinical supervision: A competency-based approach*. APA.

Fredman, G., Jahan, S., Messent, P., & Uddin, Md. Z. (2018). Joining with Bangladesh at IFTA, Malaga 2017. *Context, 156*, 46–48.

Gehart, D. (2016). Reflexivity, compassion and diversity. In K. V. Hardy & T. Bobes (Eds.), *Culturally sensitive supervision and training: Diverse perspectives and practical applications*. Routledge.

Hardy, K. V. (2016). Towards the development of a multicultural relational perspective in training and supervision. In K. V. Hardy & T. Bobes (Eds.), *Culturally sensitive supervision and training: Diverse perspectives and practical applications*. Routledge.

Lawless, J. J., Gale, J. E., & Bacigalupe, G. (2001). The discourse of race and culture in family therapy supervision: A conversation analysis. *Contemporary Family Therapy, 23*, 181–197.

Messent, P. (2017). Supervision across ethnic difference: Learning of a White supervisor and manager. In J. Bownas & G. Fredman (Eds.), *Working with embodiment in supervision: A systemic approach*. Routledge.

Papadopoulos, R. (2017). *Keynote at the International Systemic Research Conference*. Heidelberg.

Pendry, N. (2012). Race, racism and systemic supervision. *Journal of Family Therapy, 34*(4), 403–418.

Pendry, N. (2017). The construction of racial identity: Implications for clinical supervison. In J. Bownas & G. Fredman (Eds.), *Working with embodiment in supervision: A systemic approach*. Routledge.

Soheilian, S. S., Inman, A. G., Klinger, R. S., Isenberg, D. S., & Kulp, L. E. (2014). Multicultural supervision: Supervisees' reflections on culturally competent supervision. *Counselling Psychology Quarterly, 27*(4), 379–392.

Watson, M. F. (2016). Supervision in Black and White: Navigating cross-racial interactions in the supervisory process. In K. V. Hardy & T. Bobes (Eds.), *Culturally sensitive supervision and training: Diverse perspectives and practical applications*. Routledge.

8

A Child-Friendly Supervision: Inviting Children to Participate

Øyvind Kvello

Introduction: Strengthening Children's Position

Children (0–18 years old) are often left out when important decisions of their concern are made. Studies show that children seldom are described in records. If they are described, it is usually in the third person, often through the eyes of adults, e.g., parents, teachers, general practitioners, etc. This seems to be the rule internationally across different kind of services for children and families, e.g., child units in somatic hospitals, psychiatric units, child protection services, low threshold offer, etc. (Cossar et al., 2014; van Bijlevald et al., 2020).

Ø. Kvello (✉)
Department of Education and Lifelong Learning, Norwegian University of Science and Technology, Trondheim, Norway
e-mail: oyvind.kvello@ntnu.no

A supervisor of services for children and families can counteract the practice of children being left out where decisions are made. Supervisors can at least work in three ways: (1) to ask the professionals for the child's opinion and make them curious on the child's perspectives, (2) strengthening mentalization of the professional and (3) helping the professionals to develop skills in talking with children.

The Child's Opinion

Hopefully, supervisors ask professionals for children's perspectives. My experience as supervisor is that even if the professionals on daily basis work with children, when presenting cases, they tend to present a lot of information about the parents before presenting the child. When professionals present cases, as a supervisor it could be fruitful to ask them to start with presenting the child to underline the point that when we know the child one can understand what kind of care they need and their developmental conditions. This is in line with the children's right to participate:

1. States Parties shall assure to the child who is capable of forming his or her own views the right to express those views freely in all matters affecting the child, the views of the child being given due weight in accordance with the age and maturity of the child.
2. For this purpose, the child shall in particular be provided the opportunity to be heard in any judicial and administrative proceedings affecting the child, either directly, or through a representative or an appropriate body, in a manner consistent with the procedural rules of national law. (The Convention on the Rights of the Child, 1989, article 12)

Sometimes professionals can represent the child's perspective, but some children refuse to talk with professionals, or they have extensive communication problems. Professional can hold a child perspective, e.g., the choices children of same age and in same situations have taken, based on empirical research, or rooted in ethical considerations.

Supervisors can help professionals to put diligence in inviting children and make it as easy as possible for them to express themselves. If children cannot or will not talk with professionals, supervisors have an important role to help professionals to use experience and empirical research as well as legal aspects. It is difficult to form children's perspectives, it is easy for professionals to be misled by biases and personal hang-ups, so it is wise to gather several professionals to be sure to take a broad perspective on what could be a child perspective.

Strengthening the Mentalization

Mentalization consists of three dimensions: (1) empathy in others, (2) self-understanding (mindfulness) and (3) self-observation, i.e., seeing oneself through the eyes of other people. Mentalization is one of the most important personality traits for people in general, as well as for professionals to fully understand clients, and supervisors to understand those supervised. The essence of mentalization is to keep in mind other's mind.

Supervisors can encourage professionals to keep children in mind when making decisions and realize children's voices to have an impact. It is all about empowering children, and the way to fulfil this is that professionals stimulate each other's mentalization through cooperation, as mentalization develops by exercise.

Skills in Talking to Children

Supervisors can encourage professionals to develop their skills in talking with children. Professionals' conversations with younger children could be challenging, at least those younger than six years of age (Bishop, 2014; Poole et al., 2014). But, from four years of age children can talk about what they like to do and what they dislike, as well as activities they do when spending time together with their parents. Children's competence to participate in professional conversations relies heavily on their cognitive and language capacity. The younger children are, the more they are in the need of the professionals' use of facilitation and clues to remember and express themselves. Talking to children is often a matter of learning by doing, because it is difficult to fully learn it by reading books.

Learning by experience could start with supervising the professionals in what kind of questions they should try to use and what kind of questions they better avoid using: children are most at ease and talks most vividly on open questions (Ahern et al., 2015; Andrews et al., 2016; Berg et al., 2019). The information children give on open questions is mainly correct and detailed. Therefore, there is an overwhelming amount of research confirming that heavily use of open questions are the best way to make sure that children participate, as well as in investigative conversations.

Professionals can use focused questions, in order to solve any misunderstandings or getting details after the use of open questions (Stolzenberg et al., 2019). One should avoid using focused questions at the beginning of dialogues, and only used in connection to open questions.

Professionals should be restrictive in using forced-choice questions or "yes"-"no"-questions (London et al., 2017), and avoid using leading (LaPuglia et al., 2014), and suggestive questions (Andrews & Lamb, 2016). Especially children under the age of eight years of age are receptive to leading and suggestive questions (Andrews & Lamb, 2016; Otgaar et al., 2018). Use of these four questions leads to information of poor quality and is almost useless and cannot be viewed as children's participation.

Children often are most relaxed when they can fiddle with objects when talking with professionals, or they can draw (Andersen & Kjærulf, 2003). Drawing is for many children stress reducing (Einarsdottir et al., 2009; Pipe & Salmon, 2009). If they want to draw, it is important not to put pressure on them to draw something from what the conversation is all about, but let them draw whatever they want to. After drawing, the children should be invited to talk about what they have drawn. Professionals should absolutely stay away from interpretating of the children's drawings, as the interpretations are strongly personal biased. By drawing, children often present important information about themselves (Gernhardt et al., 2016), and it helps them to remember more details to put into their narratives (Gentle et al., 2014). Drawings does not only help children to relax, remember and express more details, it also helps professionals to be good at asking open questions instead of questions of poor quality (Gross et al., 2009; Patterson & Hayne, 2011). Supervisors should encourage and advice professionals to invest in a toolbox to help children of different ages to express themselves.

Supervisors can also remind professionals that it is difficult for children to understand time before the age of seven or eight. Actually, time understanding develops even through adolescence and early adulthood (Droit-Volet, 2013; Forman, 2015; Gosse & Roberts, 2014; Lamotte et al., 2012; Ogden et al., 2017; Zélanti & Droit-Volet, 2011).

Children tend to be overly optimistic before the age of six (Diesendruck & Lindenbaum, 2009; Lockhart et al., 2016). This includes themselves, other people's options and choices, as well as situations. Analyses of children's answers must always see this in the light of their tendencies to be overly optimistic.

Before the age of seven children can answer nonsense-questions, like: "Is red heavier than blue?", "Is stop stronger than go?" or "Is milk bigger than water?". This tendency seems to be of higher incidence among children from western societies than children from other cultures (London et al., 2017). Probably is this all about that children of individualistic (western) cultures are expected to be sure, and that doubts are signs of weakness.

There is on average 30% overlap between answers when children are asked the same questions several times. While some young children tend to think that the professional did not like the answer if asked the same questions several times, they can make up a new answer. Children from the age of seven years tell different but not incorrect details when questions are repeated (Andrews & Lamb, 2014; Poole, 2016; Waterhouse et al., 2016). The concept of reminiscence involves the tendency to remember new information when talking about a topic several times. The concept of hypermnesia denotes the tendency to remember more details when talking about the same issue several times (Erdelyi & Becker, 1974). To talk oneself into the topic helps people to remember (La Rooy et al., 2005). Keeping this in mind, it seems to be wise to encourage professionals to start talking to children to gain experience which often make professionals so curious that they feel like seeking knowledge.

As supervisor it is important to underline the importance of hearing children and encourage social workers to develop their skills in professional conversations with children. Lack of competence cannot be an excuse for not include children's perspectives. The best is to either study conversations with children or ask for supervision as professionals develop skills in communication with children.

The Content of Hearing Children's Voices

Supervisors should be aware that informing children and let them express themselves hardly is participating. When children are allowed to discuss and negotiate (the right to influence and the right to participate) as well as decide, they are participators (Fig. 8.1). Supervisors should hold these standards when supervising professionals to underline how common practice have to change to fulfil children's right to participate.

On a concrete level a "quality control list" of children's participating could include these steps:

1. To use suitable rooms that has furniture and equipment that is suitable for children.
2. Letting children have access to use communication tools, as the possibility for drawing, figures, dolls, stuffed animals like bears,

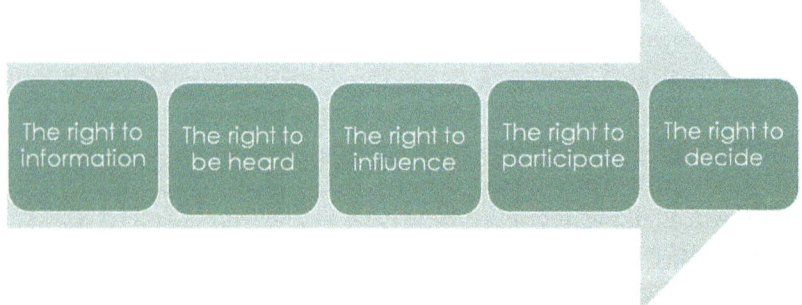

Fig. 8.1 Different degrees of participation

dogs, cats, etc. The older the child is, the less they need communication tools.
3. The form and length of conversations is adjusted to the child's age, cognitive capacity and language skills, as well as the conversation content.
4. Children are given sufficient information and necessary explanation in order to support the child to choose among options or to express themselves.
5. The information given should be non-directive and nuanced.
6. The professionals who inform the child should be neutral and they should not have preferences for what the child should express or what options they choose.
7. Sometimes it is ethical important to limit the number of options in order to make sure that children choice are in line with the law, governmental decisions, standards for the unit, etc.
8. Children should be given time to make up their mind, which means that they should not be stressed to expedite a decision.
9. Children are supported during the time they need to make up their mind, i.e., to give supplementary information, repeat given information, assure them that their opinions are important and that they are participating.
10. Professionals check out that the children are understood correctly by summarizing at the ends of the talks what they think the child have expressed and letting children confirm, correct or add information.
11. It rests a great responsibility on professionals that have heard the child's perspective to refer to what children have told where decision are taken, and work for realizing the children's opinions.
12. If the child cannot express themselves or do not want to talk with professionals, the latter is missing the child's perspective and should front children's perspective or check out if the child has conveyed their perspectives to other persons.
13. Children are given feedback on their influence/degree of participating by telling them what kind of decisions are made in accordance with the children's opinions. This is important for their self-agency and understanding of democratic processes.

Strengthening Children's Self-Agency

Letting children's voices to be heard is all about enhancing children's positions by encourage professionals to invite them to participate, and not just listen to them, but let them cooperate and sometimes decide. An important aspect of inviting children to express themselves, negotiate and make decisions is to enhance their self-agency and learn to be a member of a democratic society. Growing up means increasing influences of their lives.

As professionals should invite children to participate and thereby enhance their self-agency, supervisors can strengthen professional's self-agency by their responses on their reflections and work and encourage them to hearing the voice of children and teach them about how to talk with children for participation.

According to Bandura (2006, 2007), there are four core properties of human agency. One such property is intentionality: People form intentions that include action plans and strategies for realizing them. The second property involves the temporal extension of agency through forethought. People set themselves goals and anticipate likely outcomes of prospective actions to guide and motivate their efforts anticipatorily. A forethoughtful perspective provides direction, coherence and meaning to one's life. The third feature is self-reactiveness. According to Bandura, agents are not only planners and forethinkers, they are also self-regulators. They adopt personal standards and monitor and regulate their actions by self-reactiveness. They do things that give them satisfaction and a sense of self-worth, and refrain from actions that bring censure. The fourth feature is self-reflectiveness. People are not only agents of action, they are self-examiners of their own functioning. Through functional self-awareness they reflect on their personal efficacy, the soundness of their thoughts and actions, the meaning of their pursuits, and make corrective adjustments if necessary. During childhood, these four cornerstones of human agency are developing in ingenious patterns, but these dimensions are not fully developed before early adulthood (Bandura, 1986).

According to the concept of human agency, belief in one's efficacy is a key personal resource in self-development, successful adaptation and change. It operates through its impact on cognitive, motivational, affective and decisional processes. Efficacy beliefs affect whether individuals think optimistically or pessimistically, in self-enhancing or self-debilitating ways. Such beliefs affect people's goals and aspirations, how well they motivate themselves, and their perseverance in the face of difficulties and adversity. Efficacy beliefs also shape people's outcome expectations (Bandura, 1997).

Efficacy beliefs determine how obstacles and impediments are viewed. People of low efficacy quickly give up trying, and those of high efficacy view impediments as surmountable by improvement of self-regulatory skills and perseverant effort. They stay the course in the face of difficulties and remain resilient to adversity. Efficacy beliefs affect the quality of emotional life and vulnerability to stress. Efficacy beliefs determine the choices people make at important decisional points. A factor that influences choice behaviour can profoundly affect the courses lives take by promoting certain competencies, values and lifestyles (Bandura, 1997).

Self-agency involves that children make up their minds and express these opinions. Agency is important both in private life and in professional life, for children as well as grown-ups. It is wise to be aware of the self-agency of the supervised, because it is important for the standard set by the professionals, the drive they have for professional development and how determinant they are. In the same way as supervisors support the professional's self-agency, can be a role model for the professionals how they can strengthen the children's agency, because it is important, among other things, for children to find motivation and courage to participate. At the same time enhancing children's agency should be a theme discussed on regular basis. Among the strongest influences on agency are: (1) to be appreciated, (2) encouragement, (3) praise, (4) comparisons with others and (5) mastery experiences. Regardless supervisor, professional or child, self-agency is a fundamental competence, and people are in the need of stimulation to create strong self-agency. The professionals should work for empowering children and involve them, which means enhancing children's self-agency, as well as supervisors should contribute to strengthening the professional's self-agency.

Learning Organizations

Effective changes of practice for letting children participate assume that supervisors support learning organization environment. It is the sum of knowledge and know-how on an organizational level instead on an individual basis that decisions of change of practice are made in sufficient ways.

Supervision of professional organized in groups is not just because it can be more effective and less expensive than individual supervision, but due to moderate to high degree of turnover in several services for children, youth and families, it is important to support the development of learning organizations, because the effects of supervision are amplified if it affects the organization instead of single employees.

Supervision is often about development to increase quality on an organizational level, not only personal development for the professionals. For Fiol and Lyles (1985), the learning of individuals can be translated into organizational learning once associations, cognitive systems and memories are shared. Organizational learning is the learning of the collective. As a part of organizational instead of individual learning, there is another school of thought that considers individuals in aggregate as creating organizational learning (Castaneda et al., 2018). In an organizational learning perspective, supervision of professionals is not a solitary phenomenon (Simon, 1991; Sun & Scott, 2003), but is viewed as emerging from the interactions of individuals within groups and collective behaviour. Organizational learning is the outcome of social construction. The social constructivist approach sees organizational learning as a process through which individual knowledge is transformed into collective knowledge as well as how such socially constructed knowledge influences and it is part of local knowledge. Huysman (2002) notes that this approach puts emphasis on the process through which an organization constructs knowledge and reconstructs existing knowledge, and organizational culture is the main determinant for the organizational learning process.

Supervisors can nourish learning organizations by: (1) supervise groups of professionals instead of individual supervisions, (2) encourage the employees to be creative and develop new ideas, (3) focus on learning from each other and cooperation, (4) fostering support healthy understanding of learning, (5) support mastery instead of adjustment, (6) personal and organizational development is continuous rather than temporary and (7) developing quality control routines.

Supervising often includes helping professionals to find their positions at work, support colleagues and cooperate (see Chapter 5). Supervisors can facilitate inspiring companionship with colleagues where the collective weighs more than the individual. Professionally inspiring and a good collegial unity counteracts turnover.

To hold an organization learning perspective is fundamental to succeed in changing the common practice where children are left out where decisions about them are taken, but to replace this with letting them participate. To ensure children's participation assumes that it is not each professional to decide the form or amount of the participation, but standards given for the organization. This is realized by organizational learning processes: "This is the way we do it" instead of "This is the way I do it".

An Inclusive Practice: To Keep Children in Mind

There is on time to include children where they have been left out and not allowed to decide. It does not mean that professionals should encourage children to decide when they do not see the consequences of their choice. It will be like to leave children to themselves. Sometimes it makes children more vulnerable when they are included in decision processes, i.e. when professionals give children information that stresses or hurts them but is thought to be necessary to make good choices. Professional's sometimes need supervision to make sure that children are not expressing opinions or make choices out of loyalty, fear or are manipulated instead of freely expressing their own will. In such situations children will bear heavy burdens and are not participating based on their own needs. Letting children participate assumes that professionals know when and how to protect children from negative consequences of participation, and to check out if the children feel free to express their opinions.

Concluding Remarks

There is a long tradition in excluding children from participation, a practice that has to end. Inviting children to participate means that supervisors should support the professionals in gaining competence talking with children and support the professionals in developing skills and work habits where they encourage children to express their opinions and letting them negotiate and sometimes decide. Letting children participate is all about ethics. Supervisors often play an important role to change organization to be more child friendly when it comes to participation. It is often insufficient to work on an individual level, it requires organizational learning processes. It is on an organizational level one sets the standards for how to let children participate. Supervisors could be of great value for professionals to set standards, to design quality assurance routines for concrete actions, as well as on a regular basis reflects upon ethical dilemmas connected to letting children participate in order to make sure they are not unnecessarily stressed, putted in a vulnerable position, or bearing heavy burdens for the choices they make or opinions expressed, and to discover when children express other people's opinions instead their own.

References

Ahern, E. C., Andrews, S. J., Stolzenberg, S. N., & Lyon, T. D. (2015). The productivity of wh-promts in child forensic interviews. *Journal of Interpersonal Violence, 33*(13), 2007–2015. https://doi.org/10.1177/0886260515621084.

Andersen, D., & Kjærulf, A. (2003). *Hva kan børn svare på? Om børn som respondenter i kvantitative spørgeskemaundersøgelser* [Children as respondents on quantitative questionnaires]. Socialforskningsinstituttet.

Andrews, S. J., Ahern, E. C., Stolzenberg, S. N., & Lyon, T. D. (2016). The productivity of wh- prompts when children testify. *Applied Cognitive Psychology, 30*(3), 341–349. https://doi.org/10.1002/acp.3204.

Andrews, S. J., & Lamb, M. E. (2014). The effects of age and delay on responses to repeated questions in forensic interviews with children alleging sexual abuse. *Law and Human Behavior, 38*(2), 171–180. https://doi.org/10.1037/lhb000064.

Andrews, S. J., & Lamb, M. E. (2016). How do lawyers examine and cross-examine children in Scotland? *Applied Cognitive Psychology, 30*(6), 953–971. https://doi.org/10.1002/acp.3286.

Bandura, A. (1986). The explanatory and predictive scope of self-efficacy theory. *Journal of Social and Clinical Psychology, 4*(3), 124–148. https://doi.org/10.1521/jscp.1986.4.3.359.

Bandura, A. (1997). *Self-efficacy: The exercise of control*. Freeman.

Bandura, A. (2006). Toward a psychology of human agency. *Perspectives on Psychological Science, 1*(2), 164–180. https://doi.org/10.1111/j.1745-6916.2006.00011.x.

Bandura, A. (2007). Reflections on an agentic theory of human behavior. *Tidsskrift for Norsk Psykologforening, 44*(8), 995–1004.

Bishop, D. V. M. (2014). *Uncommon understanding: Development and disorders of language comprehension in children*. Psychology Press.

Berg, R. C., Munthe-Kaas, H. M., Baiju, N., Muller, A. E., & Brurberg, K. G. (2019). *The accuracy of using openended questions in structured conversations with children: A systematic review*. Folkehelseinstituttet.

Castaneda, D. I., Manrique, L. F., & Cuellar, S. (2018). Is organizational learning being absorbed by knowledge management? A systematic review. *Journal of Knowledge Management, 22*(2), 299–325. https://doi.org/10.1108/JKM-01-2017-0041.

Cossar, J., Brandon, M., & Jordan, P. (2014). You've got to trust her and she's got to trust you: Children's views on participation in the child protection system. *Child and Family Social Work, 21*(1), 103–112.

Diesendruck, G., & Lindenbaum, T. (2009). Self-protective optimism: Children's biased beliefs about the stability of traits. *Social Development, 18*(4), 946–961. https://doi.org/10.1111/j.1467-9507.2008.00494.x.

Droit-Volet, S. (2013). Time perception in children: A neurodevelopmental approach. *Neuropsychologia, 51*(2), 220–234. https://doi.org/10.1016/j.neuropsychologia.2012.09.023.

Einarsdottir, j, Dockett, S., & Perry, B. (2009). Making meaning: Children's perspectives expressed through drawings. *Early Child Development and Care, 179*(2), 217–232. https://doi.org/10.1080/03004430802666999.

Erdelyi, M. H., & Becker, J. (1974). Hypermnesia for pictures: Incremental memory for pictures but not words in multiple recall trials. *Cognitive Psychology, 6*(1), 159–171.

Fiol, C. M., & Lyles, M. A. (1985). Organizational learning. *Academy of Management Review, 10,* 803–813.

Forman, H. (2015). Events and children's sense of time: A perspective on the origins of everyday time-keeping. *Frontiers in Psychology, 6,* 259. https://doi.org/10.3389/fpsyg.2015.00259.

Gentle, M., Powell, M. B., & Sharman, S. J. (2014). Mental context reinstatement or drawing: Which better enhances children's recall of witnessed events and protects against suggestive questions? *Australian Journal of Psychology, 66*(3), 158–167. https://doi.org/10.1111/ajpy.12040.

Gernhardt, A., Keller, H., & Rübelling, H. (2016). Children's family drawings as expressions of attachment representations across cultures: Possibilities and limitations. *Child Development, 87*(4), 1069–1078. https://doi.org/10.1111/cdev.12516.

Gherardi, S. (2000). Practice-based theorizing on learning and knowing in organizations. *Organization, 7,* 211–223.

Gosse, L. L., & Roberts, K. P. (2014). Children's use of a «time line» to indicate when events occurred. *Journal of Police and Criminal Psychology, 29*(1), 36–43. https://doi.org/10.1007/s11896-013-9118-x.

Gross, J., Hayne, H., & Drury, T. (2009). Drawing facilitates children's reports of factual and narrative information: Implications for educational contexts. *Applied Cognitive Psychology, 23*(7), 953–971. https://doi.org/10.1002/ACP.1518.

Huysman, M. (2002). *Organizational learning and communities of practice: A social constructivist perspective.* Retrieved March 5, 2010 from http://apollon1.alba.edu.gr/OKLC2002/athens2.pdf.

Lamotte, M., Izaute, M., & Droit-Volet, S. (2012). Awareness of time distortions and its relation with time judgment: A metacognitive approach. *Consciousness and Cognition, 21*(2), 835–842. https://doi.org/10.1016/j.concog.2012.02.012.

La Rooy, D., Pipe, M. & Murray, J. E. (2005). Reminiscence and hypermnesia in children's eyewitness memory. *Journal of Experimental Child Psychology, 90*(3), 235–254.

LaPuglia, J. A., Wilford, M. M., Rivard, J. R., Chan, J. C. K., & Fisher, R. P. (2014). Misleading suggestions can alter later memory reports even following a cognitive interview. *Applied Cognitive Psychology, 28*(1), 1–9. https://doi.org/10.1002/acp.2950.

Lockhart, K. L., Goddu, M. K., & Keil, F. C. (2016). Overoptimism about future knowledge: Early arrogance? *The Journal of Positive Psychology*. https://doi.org/10.1080/17439760.2016.1167939.

London, K., Hall, A. K., & Lytle, N. E. (2017). Does it help, hurt, or something else? The effect of a something else response alternative on children's performance on forced-choice questions. *Psychology, Public Policy, and Law*, *23*(3), 281–289. https://doi.org/10.1037/law0000129.

Ogden, R. S., Samuels, M., Simmons, F., Wearden, J. & Montgomery, C. (2017). The differential recruitment of short[1]term memory and executive functions during time, number, and length perception: An individual differences approach. *The Quarterly Journal of Experimental Psychology*, *71*(3), 657–669. https://doi.org/10.1080/17470218.2016.1271445.

Otgaar, H., Howe, M. L., Merckelbach, H., & Muris, P. (2018). Who is the better eyewitness? Sometimes adults but at other times children. *Current Directions in Psychological Science*, *27*(5), 378–385. https://doi.org/10.1177/0963721418770998.

Patterson, T., & Hayne, H. (2011). Does drawing facilitate older children's reports of emotionally laden events? *Applied Cognitive Psychology*, *25*(1), 119–126. https://doi.org/10.1002/acp.1650.

Pipe, M.-E., & Salmon, K. (2009). Dolls, drawing, body diagrams, and other props: Role of props in investigative interviews. In K. Kuehnle & M. Connell (Eds.), *The evaluation of child sexual abuse allegations: A comprehensive guide to assessment and testimony* (pp. 365–395). Wiley.

Poole, D. A. (2016). *Interviewing children: The science of conversation in forensic contexts*. Washington, DC: The Ameri can Psychological Association.

Poole, D. A., Dickinson, J. J., & Brubacher, S. P. (2014). Sources of unreliable testimony from children. *Roger Williams University Law Review*, *19*, 382–410.

Simon, H. A. (1991). Bounded rationality and organizational learning. *Organization Science*, *2*, 125–134.

Stolzenberg, S. N., Williams, S., McWilliams, K., Liang, C., & Lyon, T. D. (2019). The utility of direct questions in eliciting subjective content from children disclosing sexual abuse. *Child Abuse and Neglect*. https://doi.org/10.1016/j.chiabu.2019.02.014.

Sun, P., & Scott, J. (2003). Exploring the divide – Organizational learning and learning organizations. *The Learning Organization*, *10*(4), 202–215.

van Bijleveld, G. G., Bunders-Aelen, J. F. G., & Dedding, C. W. M. (2020). Exploring the essence of enabling child participation with child protection services. *Child and Family Social Work, 25*(2), 286–293. https://doi.org/10.1111/cfs.12684.

Waterhouse, G. F., Ridley, A. M., Bull, R., La Rooy, D. & Wilcock, R. (2016). Dynamics of repeated interviews with children. *Applied Cognitive Psychology, 30*(5), 713–721. https://doi.org/10.1002/acp.3246.

Zélanti, P., & Droit-Volet, S. (2011). Cognitive abilities explaining age-related changes in time perception of short and long durations. *Journal of Experimental Child Psychology, 109*(2), 143–157. https://doi.org/10.1016/j.jecp.2011.01.003.

9

Safety and Self-Care of the Supervisor

Arlene Vetere

Introduction

> We are open to absorbing profound loss, hurt and mistrust from our clients but also to the stimulation of those states, present in us all. (Berger, 2001)

I open this chapter with Hatti Berger's poignant words. She wrote this while working for the London Underground staff counselling service, in which she explores the double-sided nature of the emotional impacts in our therapeutic work. When we include the supervisor in the above quotation, we might wonder about the triple sided nature of the impacts for the supervisor, as they live within, and reflect on, the triangle of supervisor-therapist-client and their respective interlocking contexts of

A. Vetere (✉)
VID Specialized University, Oslo, Norway

influence. There are many sources of emotional resonance in our therapeutic and supervisory work, so the key questions I shall address here centre around the development of resiliency and receptivity for practitioners, supervisors and their teams that help in sustaining supportive working contexts.

As therapists and supervisors, our practice is complex and demanding. We work in contexts of cultural and ideological diversity with our clients and colleagues within a multi-layered spirit of practice in modern social and healthcare systems. In my experience, good supervision is fundamental to the maintenance of both professional vitality and care of self and others. Clear communication, collaborative practices and warmly attuned engagement are recognized to be common factors in recovery and healing. We can see there are many similarities between therapy and supervision processes, not least in the significance of the working alliance as the vehicle for change. However, the supervisory relationship can differ in one very significant way. It can be very long lasting indeed and founded in a tried, committed and deeply trusting process. I have been supervising many practitioners for over ten years and some for nearly twenty. The continuing development of interpersonal trust in the supervisory relationship enables us to explore the felt sense of safety in our work and thus the deeper recesses of experience. For example, we may discuss important life challenges and changes with our supervisors, such as career development and changing our jobs, and the shifting nature of the balance between care of others and care of ourselves. It has taken me a long time to realize that one of the most helpful questions I can ask of a new supervisee is: 'What is there in your early attachment history, that you want me to know about, that will help us understand when you have difficulty in your therapeutic work?' This discussion allows us to anticipate possible resonance in the therapeutic work, and in the supervisory relationship, with the supervisee. Thus if the supervisee is ever feeling hopeless, helpless or otherwise stuck in their work, we might zoom in and recognize a resonance, and then zoom out. This recognition and connection to their history might be sufficient to free them up to think and feel in a more integrated and reflective way about their client and their work together. And of course, the same question can always be asked in the supervision of supervision.

In supervision, we have time and space to reflect on our reasons for doing both therapeutic and supervisory work, and to explore development and change in relation to the meanings our work holds for us. Sometimes we question why we continue to do this work, and we may need particular support from our supervisor at times of crisis when too much may be demanded of us (Hanks & Vetere, 2016). Nevertheless supervision is always a context for reflection on changes in our work-related experiences and the fit between current demands and resources and personal and professional development.

Supervision and the Arousal of Anxiety

Supervision and consultation to our therapeutic practice occurs at all stages of our career from training to post-qualification and later on to the supervision of our supervision. Our work is subject to scrutiny, critique and possibly surveillance with implied and specific ideas about what constitutes good practice. We are expected to explore our mistakes, prejudices, and our successes, and to learn—and in order to learn we need to be relatively calm and to feel safe. The discourses and practices in supervision processes may vary with the purpose of supervision, for example, training, line management, performance management, personal and professional development, and so on, but in this chapter, I wish to focus on the context and relationships that enable the development of a felt sense of safety for all. What has to happen in the moment, and over time, that we feel able to take the necessary emotional and practical risks to trust others and thus do our best to support those in our communities who need our assistance? I shall start to address this question by exploring the relationship between empathy and the supervisory alliance.

Empathy and the Supervisory Alliance

Much less has been written about the place of empathy in the supervisory alliance than in the therapeutic alliance and even less has been written about how we do empathy rather than how we feel it or conceptualize it (Vetere, 2017). Interpersonal trust grows when the other is accessible, responsive and engaged with us. We need to be seen and heard. Good listening soothes us, it helps us tolerate ambiguity and to calm down when we are worried or anxious about our work. Good listening supports reflection and self-reflexivity. The listener listens without formulating their reply while we are talking—they offer connection, affirmation, and assistance before making a challenge if needed.

Supervisors offer comfort in response to difficult emotional experiences and assist in exploring the meaning of powerful human interactions within the therapeutic triangle and our working relationships. This makes it safe to explore and clarify our experiences, so that we may integrate thought, feeling, action and intention. This is coherence. Working slowly to assist the development of understanding and perceptual flexibility, and summarizing what we hear as supervisors, helps the supervisee pause, reflect and thus process experience. In group-based supervision, as supervisors we affirm and model acceptance of all experiences. Each supervisee can also act as peer supervisor for the others, such that roles multiply and intertwine in ways that can be both empowering and fostering of competence. Both listeners and speakers become learners and listening to others means listening to oneself. In this context of safety, we are helped to organize and integrate experience in such a way that we know how to go on.

Attentiveness and Attunement

What the supervisor and the supervisee can create in their relationship offers a model of what can happen in therapy. While this is very important for trainees, it remains of crucial importance for all stages in our careers as psychotherapists and supervisors. When I prepare to meet a supervisee, I wonder how they will be. I always ask, 'How are you?' This is not a polite question as such, it is a direct and focused enquiry about the well-being of the supervisee. And when a supervisee meets me, they anticipate this question and this is where we begin. Sometimes a supervisee might be feeling confused and/or overwhelmed with work and life events and they will not know how they are! But they know that this is where we shall start our meeting.

According to Bowlby, autonomy and dependency are different aspects of the attachment process (1973). Thus we can find strength in connection—knowing we can rely on ourselves and that we can rely on others. Exploration and risk taking can be seen as a flow in which we take steps forward and explore while able to return for support, affirmation and gentle challenge. In our moments of meeting, emotional sensitivity and attunement support the monitoring of arousal and our affective rhythms (Schore & Schore, 2008). Resilience in the face of stress and novelty is helped by our capacity for non-conscious interactive regulation in our close relationships. It is when we notice a discrepancy that such monitoring becomes conscious, for example, between what is said and the way it is said, or taking our bodily reactions seriously. The regulatory processes of synchrony between feeling states and non-verbal expression in the supervisory exchanges co-create growth enhancing contexts for all participants. In both supervision and practice we ask, 'how do we learn to work with what is communicated that may not be easily expressed with words?' It needs to be safe to stumble, to search for the words for not yet worded feelings and sensations, to hesitate and to express our doubts, ambiguities and anxieties—where certainty and uncertainty are held in equal regard. Then we can lend our hearts and ears to novelty (Grover, 2017). We can feel lonely when we are not understood and emotional isolation can be traumatizing—we long to be met in a relationship where we are heard and we hear. This is compassion in action, when what is being said touches the listener and changes both the speaker and the listener. According to Castonguay et al. (2006), the essence of change is in a corrective emotional experience.

Thomas Skovolt (2001), in his research with psychotherapists, observed that a central occupational strength in the pastoral and caring professions is the capacity to stand in the shoes of the other and to be curious about the perspectives of others. He points out that such perspective taking makes the boundary regulation between the needs of self and the needs of others a more difficult task. This is often the focus in supervision, especially when we explore times of feeling overwhelmed and anxious, and times of feeling underwhelmed, cut off and distant. Bruce Wampold (2011), in his research, explores the variability between therapists within the same psychotherapeutic modality in relation to outcomes. Two of his findings that are pertinent here include the ability of the practitioner to understand, manage and regulate their own unhelpful physiological arousal during difficult moments in therapy, and to co-create a collaborative formulation with their clients—a shared understanding that makes clear to all how they might proceed in the work. In my supervision practice, I sometimes find that supervisees' experiences of unhelpful arousal and anxiety is linked to their work in more structured therapeutic models, such as Cognitive Behavioral Therapy (CBT), Dialectical Behavior Therapy (DBT) and so on, when they worry that they lack the skills to use the model. This conjoint modulation of arousal helps us know how to be in relation to others: colleagues, clients, supervisees and supervisors. Thus, supervisors can be central to, and supportive of, both these processes in their supervisees' practice. Once again we see the therapeutic triangle in action.

Supervision and Therapy: 'The Continuous Flow of Our Work...'

Thomas Skovolt and Trotter-Mathison (2011) coined the phrase, 'the continuous flow of our (therapeutic) work' and identified four phases of (a) empathic attachment, (b) active involvement, (c) felt separation and (d) renewal and recreation. I would like to suggest that these phases can sometimes describe a supervisory relationship, whether it be time limited as during training, for example, or limited by a supervisor or practitioner changing jobs or retiring. Empathic attachment involves that combination of perceptual flexibility, emotional empathy and sensitivity, and tolerance of ambiguity that promotes reflexivity, curiosity and active engagement with the work. As trust develops in the supervisory relationship, we co-create a growth enhancing context. This enables exploration of our own self-protective and defensive strategies and how they might interact within the therapeutic triangle to promote interactive repair following relationship rupture or to explain how apology restimulates remembrance of past hurts and becomes difficult to enact. As supervisors and therapists we make a commitment every day of our working lives to be present, to be focused, to be open to novel experience, and with sufficient energy to receive and welcome others, whatever else may be happening in our lives. I never wish to underestimate the energy needed to manage our own arousal and resonances and to bring these processes into a self-reflexive awareness, whether we are inclined to become over-aroused and overwhelmed in response to threat, or, on the other hand, to try to down-regulate our arousal and to dismiss our emotional reactivity (Dallos & Vetere, 2009). In many ways this working commitment is taken for granted—an unsung marvel, so to say, that the systemic literature has paid little attention to over the years, leaving this research to be conducted primarily by individually focused practitioners (Vetere & Stratton, 2016).

Professional loss is described by the supervisor's notion of felt separation—for example, the poignancy and pleasure of seeing trainees graduate and embrace their careers and then greeting the next cohort, or of saying farewell to supervisees who have become close colleagues. This process while sad is also energizing as we anticipate new experiences. In my own working life, Jan Cooper and I established 'Reading Safer Families' over 26 years ago—an independent family violence intervention service (Cooper & Vetere, 2005). We worked together with every couple and family we met, alternating our roles of lead therapist and in-room consultant. Our working relationship brought the reflecting process into the room with our clients so that all could take turns as listeners, speakers and observers. Jan and I received supervision outside of the direct therapeutic work, and of course, offered consultation and supervision in the room with our clients. This way of working helped us both to be bold in the work, and to address the concerns, fears, responsibilities and moral dilemmas inherent in hurting the people we live with and say we love.

A few years ago, Jan retired from therapeutic practice. At the time of this writing, we still train and supervise others together, but I would say I have not forgiven her for retiring! Jan knows I say this, and it is partly tongue in cheek, of course, because I wish her well in her retirement, but the loss of her, to me in the work I do, is profound and I feel her loss at every representational level: in my thinking, feeling, intending and acting as a therapist and as a co-supervisor. To say that we love our colleagues is not to exaggerate—it is felt in their responsiveness to us, their engagement with our concerns, their consistency and our reciprocity. It is a form of attachment-based responding grounded in a felt sense of mutual safety.

Different endings are always possible. There is less research on endings than on beginnings so that we know less about supervisors' and practitioners' experiences of loss in their work. As I describe above, I have been fortunate that the ending of my co-supervisory relationship with Jan has been planned, paced and flexibly managed with time for both of us to adjust. It was not an abrupt ending and/or without explanation, as some endings can be. It was not an opaque ending where we think a meeting has gone well, but the other does not return, and/or the feedback is unclear as to what happened. Some endings are complex and make learning from errors of judgement difficult, particularly if we fear failure and avoid confronting an experience that has been unclear, confusing or troubling. In these moments we see the signal importance of supervision for supervisors (Fossli & Michaelsen, 2017). As Bowlby (1973) observed, we are at our happiest and able to use our talents to the best advantage when we know there is at least one other trusted person who will come to our aid should difficulties arise.

Endings can be new beginnings. For clients, endings can hold the promise and confidence to navigate new life experiences without needing so much to fall back on 'old' self-protective strategies. For supervisees, endings can hold the promise of further professional development and trust in the processes of learning. For supervisors, endings can energize the development of new supervisory relationships, in mutually reinforcing and caring ways. Such endings renew and restore us, in all our professional roles, as we work for the benefit of others in our communities.

Conclusion

In this chapter, I hope I have shown how professional and team resiliency is supported and strengthened through trust and connection. Modern attachment theory, as a theory of both arousal regulation and integrative reflexivity, points the way to the development of the secure base in supervision process and practice. Systemic theory offers an understanding of the intersection of power and control in relationships and the relative influence of context and diversity with the need for safety and protection, for all participants in the therapeutic triangle. For me, as a supervisee, supervision has contributed to my understanding of tumult in the workplace and thus helped me navigate some complex and demanding circumstances, both internal and external. In short, it has kept me working!

References

Berger, H. (2001). Trauma and the therapist. In T. Spiers (Ed.), *Trauma: A practitioner's guide to counselling*. Brunner Routledge.
Bowlby, J. (1973). *Separation: Anxiety and anger*. Basic Books.
Castonguay, L. G., Constantino, M. J., & Holtforth, M. C. (2006). The working alliance: Where are we and where should we go? *Psychotherapy: Theory Research, Practice, Training, 43*, 271–279.
Cooper, J., & Vetere, A. (2005). *Domestic violence and family safety: A systemic approach to working with violence in families*. Wiley.
Dallos, R., & Vetere, A. (2009). *Systemic therapy and narratives of attachment: Applications in clinical settings*. Routledge.
Fossli, G., & Michaelsen, H. C. (2017). When the supervision process falters and breaks down: Pathways to repair. In A. Vetere & J. Sheehan (Eds.), *Supervision of family therapy and systemic practice: Systemic and reflective approaches with individuals, couples, families, teams and organisations*. Springer.
Grover, T. (2017). The supervisor's power and moments of learning. In A. Vetere & J. Sheehan (Eds.), *Supervision of family therapy and systemic practice: Systemic and reflective approaches with individuals, couples, families, teams and organisations*. Springer.
Hanks, H., & Vetere, A. (2016). Working at the extremes: The impact on us of doing the work. In A. Vetere & P. Stratton (Eds.), *Interacting selves: Systemic solutions for personal and professional development in counselling and psychotherapy*. Routledge.
Schore, J., & Schore, A. (2008). Modern attachment theory: The central role of affect regulation in development and treatment. *Clinical Social Work Journal, 36*, 9–20.

Skovolt, T. (2001). *The resilient practitioner: Burnout prevention and self care strategies for counselors, therapists, teachers and health professionals*. Allyn and Bacon.

Skovolt, T., & Trotter-Mathison, M. (2011). *The resilient practitioner: Burnout prevention and self care strategies for counselors, therapists, teachers and health professionals* (2nd ed.). Routledge.

Vetere, A. (2017). An attachment narrative approach to systemically informed supervision practice. In A. Vetere & J. Sheehan (Eds.), *Supervision of family therapy and systemic practice: Systemic and reflective approaches with individuals, couples, families, teams and organisations*. Springer.

Vetere, A., & Stratton, P. (Eds.). (2016). *Interacting selves: Systemic solutions for personal and professional development in counselling and psychotherapy*. Routledge.

Wampold, B. (2011). *Qualities and actions of effective therapists*. Continuing Education in Psychology. Education Directorate, American Psychological Association.

Index

C

Child protection 3, 151
Children 4–6, 38, 41, 61, 69, 77, 78, 81, 83, 87, 91, 92, 151–162
Childrens participation 6, 153, 154, 156, 158, 160–162
Content ethics 4, 56–58, 64, 68, 69
Coordinated Management of Meaning (CMM) 33–36, 41, 112
Counselling 1, 6, 81, 86, 89, 111, 167
Creativity 92, 105, 110, 115–117
Culture 4–6, 12, 33, 37, 40, 57, 63, 72, 107, 115, 119, 120, 122, 123, 128–130, 132, 134–137, 139–141, 144, 145, 147, 155, 160
Curiousity 6

E

Ethics 4, 21, 30, 31, 55–61, 63, 64, 66–73, 129, 162
Everyday ethics 71

G

GgRRAAAACCEEESSSS 4, 40–43

I

Intercultural 122–124, 126–129, 141, 144, 145

L

Learning organizations 6, 160

M

Mental health 3

Motivational Interviewing (MI) 5, 78, 86

P
Pluralistic 3, 9–12, 18, 21, 22
Power 4, 55, 56, 60, 61, 66, 68, 71–73, 80–82, 84, 87, 88, 90, 122, 142, 175
Process ethics 4, 57, 64, 69
Psychotherapy 1, 3, 89

R
Reflexivity 50, 66, 67, 112–114, 172, 174
Relational processes 1, 2, 9, 56, 68, 78, 92
Relational responsibility 4, 55, 56, 59, 68, 70, 73, 115, 116, 122
Relational self 3, 25

S
Safety 6, 109, 167–170, 174, 175
Self-care 6

Self-reflexivity 43, 121, 135, 136, 141, 147, 170
Social construction 3, 9–11, 13, 15, 17, 18, 20, 64, 69, 160
Social control 4, 72, 77, 85, 87, 88, 93
Stuck 5, 73, 103–106, 108, 111, 114–116, 168
Stuck-ness 5, 103, 104, 107, 111–117
Supervision 1–6, 9–11, 13–15, 17–19, 22, 25, 27, 29–32, 34, 35, 40–42, 55, 56, 58, 63–65, 69, 70, 72, 73, 77–80, 89–91, 93, 103, 104, 106, 110, 111, 115–117, 120–131, 133–136, 138, 139, 141–145, 147, 151, 156, 160, 161, 168–175
Systemic 3–5, 11, 13, 26, 30, 33, 107, 108, 111, 133–136, 138, 139, 141, 147, 148, 173, 175

T
Therapeutic alliance 88, 109, 169
Therapeutic relationship 3, 14, 27, 42

GPSR Compliance
The European Union's (EU) General Product Safety Regulation (GPSR) is a set of rules that requires consumer products to be safe and our obligations to ensure this.

If you have any concerns about our products, you can contact us on

ProductSafety@springernature.com

In case Publisher is established outside the EU, the EU authorized representative is:

Springer Nature Customer Service Center GmbH
Europaplatz 3
69115 Heidelberg, Germany

www.ingramcontent.com/pod-product-compliance
Ingram Content Group UK Ltd.
Pitfield, Milton Keynes, MK11 3LW, UK
UKHW020405080825
461681UK00003B/21